MW00967474

You Can
Prevent Heart Attack

Coronary Heart Disease (CHD) is perhaps one of the most dreaded diseases in the world—partly because of the sheer magnitude of the problem and partly because it can kill dramatically and without warning. Yet much of this epedemic is self made.

What we eat, the amount and types of dietary fats we consume, how we live, what stress we load on ourselves and the environment, how much we exercise are important causal factors in heart problems. There may occasionally be other lesser known predisposing factors; yet the preventive potential of this disease cannot be over-emphasized.

Adequate precautions *can* prevent heart attak to a very large degree. The do's and don'ts prescribed by the author, are simple preventive measures which would help keep your heart in mint condition and away from the dread of a potential heart attack.

The author also takes the reader on a unique journey through the heart, explaining how it functions. He discusses the results of the latest researches in CHD and the trends in its surgical management. There are key facts on combating obesity, hypertension and the twin evils of smoking and cholestrol.

"Based on pains taking research and long experience, the book bears a stamp of authority...the author's easy style makes the book imminently readable and informative."

Pioneer

The Author

Dr. O.P. Jaggi is not only a renowned physician and a medical scientist of international standing, but is also a crusader in the field of demystifying medicine and medical facts for the common man. He firmly believes in the concept of preventive medicine and, therefore, in explaining medical facts. His books on health-care namely *You Can Prevent Heart Attack; To Drink or Not to Drink; All About Malaria : Causes, Prevention and Cure; All About Allopathy, Homeopathy, Ayurveda, Unani and Nature Cure; Mental Tension and Its Cure* (all available in Orient Paperbacks), are immensely popular. During his professional life extending over 30 years, he has travelled widely & studied health problems under different environments. He has been Senior Consultant Physician to the Government of Nigeria. Also he has been Dean, Faculty of Medical Sciences, University of Delhi and Director, V. Patel Chest Institute, Delhi. Currently he is the head of the Clinical Research Department, V. Patel Chest Institute, University of Delhi. He is the President of Foundation for Total Health-Care and President of Self-Care for Asthma Foundation.

You Can Prevent
Heart Attack

Dr. O.P. Jaggi
M.B.B.S., M.D., Ph.D.
F.C.C.P.(USA), F.A.C.A.(USA)
F.R.A.S.(London)

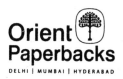

Orient
Paperbacks

DELHI | MUMBAI | HYDERABAD

www.orientpaperbacks.com

ISBN 13: 978-81-222-0097-3
ISBN 10: 81-222-0097-4

1st Published 1975
Revised & Enlarged Edition 1984
15th Printing 2011

You Can Prevent Heart Attack

© O.P. Jaggi, 1984

Cover design by Vision Studio

Published by
Orient Paperbacks
(A division of Vision Books Pvt. Ltd.)
5A/8, Ansari Road, New Delhi-110 002

Printed and bound at
Saurabh Printers Pvt. Ltd., New Delhi

Cover Printed at
Ravindra Printing Press, Delhi-110 006

Contents

Preface to the
Revised Edition

Ask a few well-informed persons over the age of 50 years: What are they afraid of the most? Four out of five would answer : Sudden death due to heart attack.

Rightly so too. Heart attack is becoming a common cause of death after the age of fifty.

It is better that people are afraid of this danger to their existence or to their health, rather than that they be foolhardy about it. Those who are afraid of it, would surely take whatever precautions or preventable measures are available against it.

Heart attack is preventable to a large extent and we know how to prevent it. We also know that by these measures people have already brought down death and ill-health caused by it.

This book deals with all these preventable measures against the heart attack. Observing these measures one can ensure long and healthy life.

Surgical treatment in a person who is at a 'high risk' or has had an heart attack or angina pectoris, is a topic of much current interest. The book describes the latest techniques in regard to 'coronary by-pass surgery', as well as the indications for undergoing such procedures and the risk involved.

The first edition of this book, written in 1974, after so many reprints and a decade in between, did need an updating because of the rapid advances being made in this important field of medicine. You will, I am sure, find the present book worthwhile and easily understandable.

O.P. Jaggi

V. Patel Chest Institute
University of Delhi
DELHI-110007

1

Introduction

From olden times, medical writers, both in India and abroad, have been aware of the fact that excessive eating and drinking, may make a man look healthy and of reddish tinge; yet in fact, he is not so. He is more prone to different diseases and to sudden death.

Sudden death was not associated with heart attack until towards the beginning of the present century. Till then the terms 'heart attack', 'coronary thrombosis' or 'cardiac infarction' were not in common use among laymen and doctors alike.

Since then, the graph of deaths due to heart attacks has been showing a steep rise. The death rate from heart attack in the United States rose from 8 per 100,000 in 1930, to 23 in 1935, to 71 in 1940, to 226 in 1952 and 290 in 1963. There has been a further tremendous increase since then. In 1985 approximately 1.5 million people suffered heart attacks in the USA, and 35 per cent of them died of it, half of the deaths occurring before the patient could reach the hospital. An additional 15 to 20 per cent of survivors died in the first year following heart attack. There is virtually an epidemic of heart attacks in the States and some other European countries.

Deaths due to heart attack are not as common in India as in some European countries; yet here also the incidence is increasing year by year. This increase is real and not due to better diagnosis. And this is certainly going to increase further, at least, for one reason since the life span of the people is increasing there are more and more older males who fall in the groups among whom heart attacks are common.

A few decades ago, coronary heart disease and subsequent heart attacks were considered as part of the ageing process. This view was essentially based upon the observations that heart attacks occurred mostly in people in the older age groups. Increasing incidence of the disease and its occurrence in younger people, even below 40 years of age, cast doubts upon the ageing process being the cause of the condition.

We now know that heart attacks are due to coronary atherosclerosis (narrowing of the coronary arteries), which process starts at a much younger age. This finding is based upon the study of the coronary and other arteries of the younger people who died either in the wars, or as a result of accidents.

Among American soldiers (average age 22 years) killed in action in the Korean War, 77 per cent were reported to have gross pathological evidence of atherosclerosis. Ten per cent exhibited far advanced disease.

Similar findings have been reported from India as well. From Lucknow in 1969, in a study based upon 300 medicolegal post-mortems, it was found that atherosclerosis of the coronary arteries was two and half times more prevalent in the males than the females. Males were completely free from it in the first two, and females in the first three decades. Over the decades, both the sexes were equally and progressively affected.

From Agra, in 1961, in a study based upon 500 medicolegal post-mortems, it was found that in the first decade 50 per cent, in the second decade 95 per cent, and after the third decade all the specimens studied showed evidence of atherosclerosis of the coronary arteries. There was a progressive rise in the extent and severity of the disease with age. This was less in females than in males for each decade from first through eighth.

Heart attacks are more common in males than in females, the ratio in many studies being about 5 to 1. Males between 40 and 60 years of age have the maximum incidence. The incidence of heart attacks in females is rising.

In the Western countries, the incidence of heart attacks is said to be more in males belonging to higher income groups. But in India, they occur equally among the rich as well as the poor. In a study from Bihar in 1971, it was reported that 40.8 per cent of all heart attacks occurred among low income groups which included farmers and manual workers. From Gujarat in 1968, the occurrence of heart attacks occupation wise was reported as follows: executives, professionals 28 per cent; clerks, teachers 23.5 per cent; manual workers 25.5 per cent; sedentary workers, shopkeepers 15.5 per cent; the retired people 7.5 per cent.

In India, heart attacks occur equally among the rural population as among the urban, with a difference, however, that among rural people, on an average, the attacks occur in the older age group as compared to the urban. This observation is contrary to the impression created by newspaper reports that heart attacks occur more commonly among urban people.

Coronary atherosclerosis starts much earlier in life; it progresses year by year, decade by decade and remains undetected, unmanifested, until it produces heart attacks.

Your Heart and the Coronaries

Your heart is as delicate as it is strong. About the size of your fist, in the chest it is enclosed in a protective covering called the pericardium. It hangs down within the chest attached to the great blood vessels, pointing downwards towards the left nipple.

The Heart

It is divided into two parts, the right and the left, by a blood-tight wall. Each part works as a separate pump for the blood it receives, and has an upper chamber, called auricle which receives blood from the large veins, and a lower chamber called ventricle which pumps out blood into the arteries.

From the right ventricle the veinous blood goes to the lungs for gaining oxygen and throwing out carbon dioxide. From the left ventricle, the arterial blood goes to the aorta to supply nourishment to all parts of the body. The ventricles are so strong that when they contract, they can squeeze out almost all the blood that is contained in them.

The steady rhythm of the heart—*lubb-dup, lubb-dup*—which can be heard by placing your ear on somebody's chest or through the doctor's stethoscope is due mainly to opening and closing of different valves inside the heart while it receives and pumps out blood. This it does, on an average, 72 times a minute, equal to your

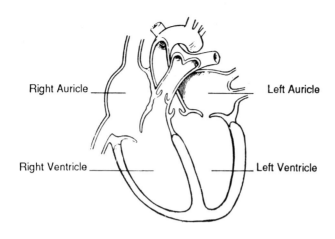

Right Auricle

Left Auricle

Right Ventricle

Left Ventricle

Fig. 1   Heart Showing Different Chambers

pulse rate. There is no man-made pump that compares in efficiency with your heart.

What causes the heart to beat? It is a kind of electrical timing apparatus called the pace-maker which normally generates about 72 times a minute, a tiny electrical impulse which sweeps over the muscle fibres, causing them to contract in an orderly fashion.

Coronary Arteries

Your heart weighs 1/200th of your weight, but it receives 1/20th of the total circulating blood for its own nourishment. This it gets not from the blood that passes through its chambers but from the coronary arteries, the two blood vessels that are the first to come off the aorta and lie embedded in the heart muscle itself. They are not much thicker than the ordinary drinking straws.

The right coronary nourishes the back of the heart and to an extent its sides. The left coronary artery is larger than the right and divides into two major branches, viz., anterior descending and posterior circumflex. These branches feed mainly the front and the left side of the heart. Each coronary artery after rising from the aorta, soon divides and subdivides into smaller and smaller branches

15

so as to reach all parts of the heart muscle. By the injection of radio-opaque materials into the coronary arteries in post-mortem specimens, it has been shown that the cross-connections (anastomoses) between the finer branches of the two coronary arteries progressively increase with age.

The anastomoses between the branches of the coronary arteries proves useful because when one branch gets blocked, the area that it served before, now receives blood supply from the other anastomosing branches. This phenomenon, however, depends upon several factors, the most important of which is the speed with which the blockade occurs; if it occurs suddenly and completely, then the anastomosing channels cannot, at once, come to the rescue.

Flaming and Schwarz of the University of Heidelburg in West Germany, showed in their experimental studies that coronary anastomoses also termed as collaterals, are able to maintain resting coronary flow after complete coronary obstruction. The functional significance of these well-developed collaterals, however, is limited, and blood flow becomes inadequate under stress conditions. In man, they found, that coronary collaterals

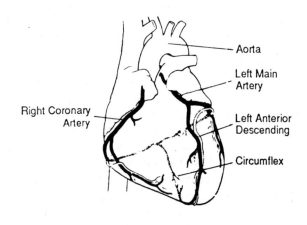

Fig. 2   **Normal Coronary Arteries**

16

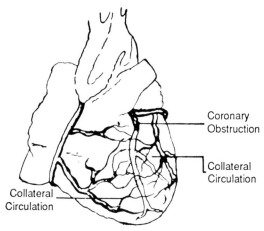

Fig. 3   Anastomosing or Collateral Coronary Vessels

compensated for the coronary obstruction only partially. Dr. Gensini of Syracuse, USA, aptly stated the case of collaterals, when he said; "I would like to illustrate the significance of the collaterals by comparing them either to a welfare cheque enabling the recipient to survive—though often at the expense of considerable financial privation, or to life boats on luxury liners. If the luxury liner sinks, the number of people that will survive will depend on the availability and the number of life boats, i.e. the collaterals: the more collaterals, the more myocardium (heart muscle) will be saved. On the other hand, however, a trip in a life boat no longer affords the luxury of the big liner and similarly the presence of collaterals will save myocardium, but often at the expense of the pain because the myocardium that will be left will be ischaemic—viable but ischaemic (short of blood supply). Hence, whenever there are more collaterals, there is more myocardium which can hurt, whereas in the absence of collaterals, there is dead myocardium, which can of course no longer hurt."

Factors Causing Coronary Narrowing

The important factors that accelerate coronary artery narrowing are:

1. Excess of fats and cholesterol in the blood
2. High blood pressure
3. Over-weight
4. Diabetes
5. Smoking

Others are male sex, family history, physical inactivity and mental stress.

Let us take these one by one.

Excess of Fats and Cholesterol

Our food consists chemically of carbohydrates, proteins, fats, vitamins, minerals and water. The fats are present in the food as such or in a combined form. Fats, that we take, are derived from animal source (*ghee* and butter) or from vegetable source (different vegetable oils and hydrogenated vegetable oil) Combined with carbohydrates and proteins, fat is present in milk, meat, eggs, lentils, cereals, nuts etc.

Fats are digested in the stomach and the intestines and absorbed from there into blood circulation. Some of them are used up to supply calorie needs of the body for performing various functions. The surplus ones are stored as such in different parts of the body.

Fats are made up of different fatty acids and glycerol. In some fatty acids, all the carbon (C) atoms are completely sandwiched between hydrogen (H) atoms, as is shown below:

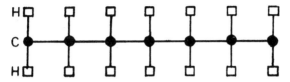

Fig. 4   Saturated Fatty Acid

It means that in them all C atoms are fully attached with or saturated with H atoms. Such fatty acids are called saturated fatty acids and when they combine with glycerol, they form solid saturated fat. The longer the sandwich of (chain of) C and H atoms, the harder the fat.

When in a fatty acid, some of the carbon atoms do not have hydrogen atoms attached to them, that fatty acid is called unsaturated. Its combination with glycerol gives rise to liquid unsaturated fats. The larger the number of unattached carbon atoms (polyunsaturated), the more liquid and unsaturated the fat.

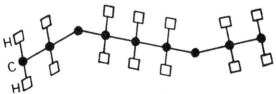

Fig. 5   Unsaturated Fatty Acid

Animal fats such as butter and *ghee* contain predominantly saturated fatty acids and hence they are solid at ordinary temperture. On the other hand, vegetable fats contain predominantly unsaturated fatty acids and hence they are liquid

19

at ordinary temperature. Most fats contain both saturated and unsaturated fats in varying proportions.

In order to solidify certain vegetable oils, they are subjected to hydrogenation of their carbon atoms. In the process, the oils are treated with hydrogen gas at a suitable temperature in the presence of a catalyser such as finely divided nickel.

Fats in the Blood: After absorption, the fats in the blood stream move about either as tiny particles of fat, or they combine with different proteins so that in this form they are soluble in the blood stream.

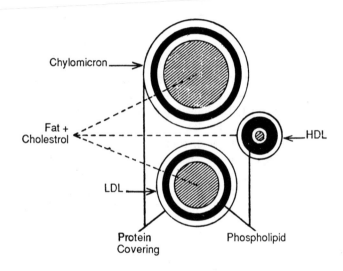

Fig. 6   Fat Particles in Blood

The particles of neutral fat in the blood chemically called triglycerides, are very tiny, about one micron in size; that is why they are called chylomicrons (chyle is the white milky product formed as a result of digestion of fats in the food). A chylomicron is about one-seventh the size of a red blood cell.

In combination with different proteins, the fats form even smaller globules than the size of chylomicrons. They are called

20

lipoproteins and according to their characteristics, they are categorized as :

1. Very Low-density Lipoproteins (VLDL);
2. Low-density Lipoproteins (LDL), previously called as beta-lipoproteins;
3. High-density Lipoproteins (HDL), previously called as alpha-lipoproteins.

The globules of these lipoproteins are made up of a core which is a mixture of fats and cholesterol. Covering the core is a layer of phospholipids, i.e. a kind of fat which contains in addition phosphoric acid and protein groups. Serving as a coating for the entire globule is an extremely thin layer of proteins. In these globules, fat dissolves the cholesterol which otherwise cannot be transported by itself as it is insoluble in the blood as such. And as pure fatty globules stick together, a layer of phospholipids and proteins removes this tendency.

If the fats and cholesterol are to be carried by the blood to their destinations in the tissues, these four substances, viz., fats, cholesterol, phospholipids and proteins must always remain linked together.

The thicker the protective coat of phospholipids, the more stable the globule. The smallest of the lipoprotein globules, HDL, has the heaviest coat and hence is the most stable.

It has been lately discovered that HDL have an inverse relationship to LDL. Epidemiologic and experimental studies have shown that high levels of HDL lessen the incidence of atherosclerosis.

Cholesterol in Food and Blood: Cholesterol is a type of fat. It is found only in animals and animal products such as milk, meat, brain, eggs etc. It is not found in vegetables or vegetable products.

Cholesterol is present in the blood and being insoluble as such, is transported alongwith other things in different lipoprotein globules.

Cholesterol is an essential constituent of our body, used in its various tissues and activities. In the brain and nervous tissue, it acts as an excellent insulator so that electrical impulses travel unhindered; without it, electrical impulses travelling in the nerves in our body would get short-circuited. Brain contains a heavy concentration of it. Cholesterol is also the source of material for the manufacture of male and female sex hormones. Yolk (yellow) of the egg has a high concentration of it.

An average adult takes about 200 to 800 mg. of cholesterol in his diet daily, depending on the amount of intake of animal fats. Cholesterol is also manufactured in the body itself by the liver from carbohydrates, proteins and fats that we take in our diet; this later amounts to 1.5 to 2.0 gm. daily. Absorption of cholesterol is aided by the fats we take and also by the bile in the intestine. The cholesterol is chiefly absorbed by the lymphatics and enters the blood stream where it is transported within the lipoprotein particles.

Cholesterol is oxidised in the body to carbon dioxide by many tissues but most actively by the liver. Some of the cholesterol is converted into steroid hormones and most of it into bile acids which are excreted in the bile. Bile acids represent the major normal degradation product of cholesterol.

The liver is the major organ concerned with cholesterol, which it can manufacture, store and destroy. By these processes, it largely determines and controls the level of blood cholesterol. The latter is maintained fairly constant by regulatory mechanisms between the absorption and synthesis of cholesterol on the one hand, and the metabolism and excretion on the other.

It has been found that the amount of cholesterol in the food has a significant effect upon the blood cholesterol level. The addition of dietary cholesterol in the form of the yellow part of the egg in healthy young men causes a significant increase in the concentration of blood cholesterol. When the yellow part of the egg is removed from the diet, level of cholesterol decreases greatly.

The intake of fat in the diet also exerts a strong influence on blood cholesterol. Short term studies have constantly shown a tendency to a fall in blood cholesterol following a diminution in the intake of fat in the diet. Populations habitually subsisting on low fat diets, as in India, certain parts of Africa etc., have a relatively low blood cholesterol levels.

An important finding in regard to fats is that the intake of unsaturated fats prevents the rise of blood cholesterol level which should otherwise occur if more fats are taken in the diet. This has been proved experimentally by feeding monkeys with more than ordinary quantity of fat, the fat being predominantly of an unsaturated variety. Clinically also, it has been observed that Eskimos who live largely on fish have lower levels of blood cholesterol; the fish fat and oil being mostly unsaturated—an exception in the case of fats derived from animal sources.

Data collected from studies all over the world indicate that the normal blood cholesterol level should be in the range of 160 to 180 mg. per 100 ml. The average blood cholesterol level in people in the United States and other affluent countries is much higher; it is somewhere between 230 and 260 mg. per 100 ml. In these affluent countries, the average blood cholesterol level has been known to have arisen during the past few decades. In Holland, it rose from 182 in 1812 to 245 mg. in 1948. In England, while the average blood cholesterol level now is lower than in the U.S.A has risen over the years; in 1925, it ranged between 150 and 200 mg. per 100 ml.

High Blood Cholesterol Level and Coronary Heart Disease: A high level of cholesterol in the blood, particularly if it is held in combination in the form of LDL globules—which are more unstable so that the cholesterol comes apart easily—leads to its deposition in the walls of the blood vessels.

Although to the naked eye, cholesterol looks waxlike, under the microscope, its real structure, as tiny sharp needles, is visible, which when deposited in the wall of the arteries irritate it severely.

Lesions in blood vessels have been produced experimentally also in rabbits, guinea pigs, hamsters, pigs, chickens and monkeys by feeding them large quantities of cholesterol or animal fat. A very high blood cholesterol level precedes the development of the lesions.

Between 1948 and 1950, when controversy about the role of cholesterol was raging, National Heart Institute in the U.S.A.,

23

started a long-term study in the town of Framingham, Massachusetts. The 5,000 people included were healthy, not sick. They lived the way they had lived all along and ate and drank as they were doing before. They, however, came for check up before the doctors every now and then and were followed up for 20 years.

By 1960, the Framingham experiment was 10 years old and some important conclusions were already available. Over a ten-year period, in the group with a cholesterol level below 200, the coronary disease occurred in 215 people. At the 200 to 220 blood cholesterol level, there were 60 cases. At the 220 to 240 level, the count was 80. At the 240 to 260 level, it was 140. And when the cholesterol level rose above 260, the number of coronary cases mounted to 200.

In the Framingham study, low HDL was a more potent lipid risk factor than the high LDL. HDL averages about 25 per cent higher in women than in men. Female sex hormones, the estrogens, tend to raise, and male sex hormones, the androgens, tend to lower HDL. In women, low HDL, particularly when associated with diabetes and obesity, markedly raises the risk of heart attacks.

The Framingham study, also showed that in men and women 35 to 44 years of age, serum cholesterol levels of 265 mg/100 ml. or over are associated with a five times higher risk of developing coronary artery disease than are levels below 220 mg/100 ml.

Similar correlations of high blood cholesterol levels with increased incidence of subsequent coronary heart disease have also been noted in other long-term studies. In all, the incidence of coronary heart disease is more particularly low when the blood cholesterol is below 200 mg/100 ml. In most of the studies, there is a sharp rise in the subsequent development of coronary heart disease in groups of individuals with blood cholesterol above 240 or 260 mg/100 ml.

In populations in which coronary heart disease has been reported to be less common, the average serum cholesterol concentration in men beyond the age of 40 is usually found to be around 180 mg/100 ml.

An interesting observation made among coronary artery disease patients is that the high blood cholesterol which they have, fluctuates widely, whereas in the normal persons the blood cholesterol level is low and it is constant. Since in the normal person, the level of blood cholesterol is close to its concentration point, deposition of cholesterol follows when there is slight elevation above normal values, resulting in atheromatous lesions.

Coronary artery disease, blood cholesterol level, and the amount of fat taken in the diet usually go hand in hand. It was found that in a Cape Town province, Bantus, the original inhabitants, obtain 16 per cent of their calories from fat, the blacks 25 per cent and the white people 40 per cent. Severe atherosclerosis and heart attacks are rare among the Bantus, fairly frequent among the Cape Province blacks and very common among the Europeans. Within each of the groups, the serum cholesterol was found to be directly related to dietary fat intake.

In Norway and other European countries, in World War II, there was a sharp reduction in morbidity and mortality from coronary heart disease due probably to the great reduction in fat and cholesterol in the diet. But no such diminution in the incidence of coronary disease occurred in Denmark despite German occupation, probably because the population continued on a high diet. Similarly when the Jews from Yemen, where they lived on a low fat diet and experienced little coronary heart disease, emigrated to Israel, where their diet became rich in fats, their serum cholesterol rose and the incidence of coronary heart disease increased significantly.

In the United States, the increased frequency of coronary heart disease has been correlated with the increase in fat calories as a per cent of total caloric intake from 31.8 per cent in 1910 to 43 per cent in 1960.

The evidence linking fatty diet, high fat content of the blood and the development of coronary artery disease can be summarized as follows:

1. Dietary cholesterol intake from 0 to 600 mg/day is closely related to plasma cholesterol levels and dietary saturated fatty acids elevate blood cholesterol levels, whereas polyunsaturated fatty acids reduce them.

2. Low-cholesterol, low saturated fat diets consistently lower blood cholesterol levels up to 10 to 20 per cent.

3. Populations with sharply lowered dietary cholesterol and saturated fatty intake, have lower blood cholesterol levels and reduced coronary heart disease.

4. Immigrants from populations having low blood cholesterol to ones in which it is high, develop cholesterol levels comparable to their host population.

5. Animal studies particularly in sub-human primates, reveal an unequivocal relationship between dietary cholesterol or saturated fat, blood cholesterol levels and atherosclerosis.

6. Partly as a result of campaigns of many organizations, principally the American Heart Association, cholesterol intake in the American population has declined since 1970, and the polyunsaturated/saturated ratio in dietary fat has increased, consequently, there has been a definite lowering trend in blood cholesterol levels of adult Americans between 1971 and 1974, compared to levels during 1960 to 1962. In the same time periods, a significant downward trend (20 per cent) in heart attack deaths occurred among persons 36 to 74 years of age.

Both high cholesterol and high triglycerides in the blood appear to be important risk factors for atherosclerosis. In adults less than 55 years of age, a cholesterol concentration greater than 200 mg/100 ml or a triglyceride concentration greater than 200 mg/100 ml, clearly indicates high fat content of the blood (hyperlipidemia) sufficient to require attention by the doctor.

If hyperlipidemia is not present, the tests need not be repeated for several years in an adult who maintains body weight and does not otherwise change in health or life-style.

High Blood Pressure (Hypertension)

Blood pressure is the pressure exerted by the blood against the walls of the arteries through which it flows. Blood pressure is highest each time the heart contracts and pumps out blood into the arteries. The reading at this time is called systolic, as systole means heart contraction. The blood pressure falls to its lowest level when the heart is relaxing. This reading is called diastolic, as diastole means heart relaxation. Both these blood pressure readings are generally recorded as the higher systolic pressure over the lower diastolic pressure, for example, 125/85.

Since there is no dividing line between normal and high blood pressure, arbitrary levels have been established to define those who have an increased risk of developing a heart or blood vessel (cardiovascular) disorder and/or will clearly benefit from medical therapy. For example, patients with a diastolic pressure greater than 90 mm Hg will have a significant reduction in disease and mortality with adequate treatment. These, then, are patients who have hypertension and who should be considered for treatment.

The level of systolic pressure is also important in assessing arterial pressure's influence on heart disease. Males with normal diastolic pressures (less than 82 mm Hg) but elevated systolic pressures (more than 158 mm Hg) have a 2 1/2 fold increase in their cardiovascular mortality rates when compared with individuals with similar diastolic pressures but whose systolic pressures are normal (less than 130 mm Hg).

Even though in an adult, hypertension is usually defined as a pressure greater than or equal to 150/90, in men under 45 years of age, a pressure greater than or equal to 130/90 mm Hg may be elevated.

Individuals can be classified as being normotensive if arterial pressure is less than levels noted above, and as having sustained hypertension if the diastolic pressure always exceeds these levels. Arterial pressure fluctuates in most persons, whether they are normotensive or hypertensive. Those who are classified as having labile hypertension are patients who sometimes have arterial pressures within the hypertensive range. These patients are often considered to have borderline hypertension.

Blood Pressure Regulation: The degree of blood pressure is regulated by various factors. The kidneys participate in this regulation. Stimuli from the nervous system and the consequent body responses, particularly the hormonal secretions of various endocrinal glands of the body are the important ones. These factors influence the blood pressure level by controlling the relaxation or contraction of the smaller arteries called arterioles. If the arterioles relax readily, the blood forced out by the heart can be accommodated in the vessels easily without heightening the blood pressure.

But if the arterioles do not relax readily then as the blood is forced into them by the heart, the pressure in them rises and remains high even in diastole. This progressive lack of relaxation of blood vessels increases blood pressure over a period of time.

In most cases of hypertension, the cause is not clearly discernible. These cases are called Idiopathic Hypertension or Essential Hypertension—though the last is a misnomer, as there is nothing essential about this high blood pressure.

Symptoms and Signs: The majority of patients with hypertension have no symptoms referable to their blood pressure elevation and will be identified only in the course of a physical examination. When symptoms do bring the patient to the physician, they fall into three categories. They are related to:

1. The elevated pressure itself.
2. The hypertensive vascular disease, and
3. The underlying disease in the case of secondary hypertension.

Though popularly considered a symptom of elevated arterial pressure, headache is characteristic only of severe hypertension; most commonly it is localized to the back of the head, is present when the patient awakens in the morning, and subsides spontaneously after several hours. Other possibly related complaints include dizziness, palpitation, and easy fatigability.

Complaints referable to vascular disease include epistaxis, blood in urine, blurring of vision owing to retinal changes, episodes of weakness or dizziness due to transient cerebral ischaemia, angina pectoris, and dyspnoea due to heart failure.

Examples of symptoms related to the underlying disease in secondary hypertension are varied.

Prognosis: Insurance statistics show that, in general, expectation of life is considerably reduced in those who have high blood pressure compared with those in whom the pressure is within the normal range. However, it does not follow that all who have high blood pressure necessarily have a bad prognosis. The condition is mild if the heart is not enlarged, the retina of the eyes (fundi) show no abnormalities and there is no protein in urine (proteinuria) or evidence of impaired kidney function. Many such patients live a life of normal span free from related illness.

On the whole, women seem to withstand hypertension better than men.

Young men, in particular, who when first seen have high diastolic pressures together with secondary manifestations in the fundi or heart, require optimal control of the blood pressure without delay.

Consequences of Hypertension: As the blood vessels do not relax to receive the blood from the heart, the heart has to work harder against this resistance. This strains the heart, so that it ultimately fails to perform its function of pumping the blood to all parts of the body.

Hypertension accelerates the process of hardening and narrowing of the blood vessels. This affects:

1. the coronary arteries leading to less blood and less oxygen being supplied to the heart muscle (myocardium) and myocardial infarction or angina;

2. cerebral arteries leading to brain strokes, and

3. renal arteries leading to less blood going through the kidney arteries for purification, and subsequent collection of waste products in the blood, the condition called uraemia.

Hypertension enhances atherogenesis by directly producing injury via mechanical stress on endothelial cells at specific high pressure sites in the arterial tree. In addition, hypertension allows more lipoproteins to be transported through the lining cells of the arteries into their walls by altering their permeability.

High blood pressure is found in about 50 per cent of men

and in about 75 per cent of women with coronary heart disease. In the Framinghām study in the USA, it was found that a blood pressure reading of greater than 160/90 mm. Hg produced a three-fold increase in risk of heart attack for men between 50 and 59 years of age, and a six-fold increase in risk for women of the same age. An increase in coronary heart disease occurred at each successive level of blood pressure, with a seven-fold increase in those with blood pressure over 180 compared to those with pressure under 120 systolic. Experimentally induced hypertension increased the serverity of atherosclerosis in laboratory animals such as rabbits, dogs, chicks and rats.

Over-weight

After age 25, a person starts gaining weight, unless he does something about the food he eats and the amount of daily activity. The reason is that, beginning at this age, the body starts to need less food because the metabolism is slowing down. The result is that he requires about 10 less calories everyday for each year that passes, and if he does not cut back by this amount, he will end up gaining about 1/2 a kilogram a year.

In general, disease and death from heart disease are higher in direct relation to the degree of over-weight. Furthermore, from data obtained in the Framingham study, it appears that obesity may accelerate atherosclerosis and its effect is more apparent before age 50. However, obesity is a disorder closely associated with other potent risk factors, i.e. hyperlipidaemia, hyperglycemia and hypertension. The relationship between obesity and atherosclerosis is thus multifaceted, and since, in practice, obesity does not occur 'independently', it is of considerable importance as a risk factor.

For people who are over-weight, the increase in death rate is calculated as follows:

Over-weight	Increase in death rate
10 per cent	13 per cent
20 per cent	25 per cent
30 per cent	40 per cent

Diabetes Mellitus

Diabetes may be defined as high level of glucose in the blood, so that some of it overflows into the urine. Usually it is due to deficiency of insulin.

It is a chronic disease and affects the utilization of carbohydrates, fats and proteins. Diabetes causes a lot of complications, an important one being the narrowing of the blood vessels called atherosclerosis. This change occurs at an earlier age in diabetics and is more extensive. The cause for this accelerated atherosclerosis is not known, although it is suggested that alterations in the ratio of high-density (HDL) to low-density lipoproteins (LDL) in plasma may play a role.

The role of glucose in atherosclerosis is poorly understood. Hyperglycemia is known to affect aortic wall metabolism.

Coronary artery disease is common in diabetics. Silent myocardial infarction is known to occur in diabetics and should be suspected whenever symptoms of left ventricular failure appear suddenly.

Diabetic patients, as a rule, suffer more heart attacks than non-diabetics, other factors remaining the same. Also, heart attacks in diabetics occur at a younger age than they do in non-diabetics.

Women who have diabetes suffer heart attacks more often so much so that in such cases the usual high ratio of heart attacks between males and females is very much lessened.

Heart attacks are also common in those people who do not yet have diabetes but their glucose metabolism on laboratory testing is found to be faulty, so that they can be labelled as pre-diabetics. In a study abroad, it was found that 46 per cent of apparently non-diabetic patients with atherosclerotic coronary heart disease had an abnormal glucose tolerance. In Kanpur, 49 per cent patients with coronary heart disease were found to have impaired glucose tolerance.

Smoking

The way cigarettes bring on heart damage is still something of a mystery, but three possible explanations are:

1. Nicotine repeatedly over-stimulates the heart.

2. The carbon monoxide absorbed into the blood takes the place of oxygen and hampers nourishment of the heart muscle and other tissues. People with angina pectoris develop the chest pain quicker if they smoke. Even being in the same room with people who are smoking may aggravate these chest pains.

3. The smoke damages the lining of the coronary arteries, allowing artery-clogging cholesterol to build up and narrow the passage ways.

Evidence that heart attacks are common among smokers is now beyond serious dispute. The risk is in proportion to the amount of tobacco smoked. This includes the age at which smoking is begun, the number of cigarettes smoked and the degree of inhalation.

The risk of heart attacks occurring at an age below 40 years and of consequent sudden death is also more among heavy smokers than among non-smokers.

Discontinuance of smoking lessens this risk, so much so that those who smoked previously but stopped later on, five years later their chances of getting heart attack had come down to the same level as those of non-smokers.

Male Sex

Heart attacks occur much more frequently among males than among females. This difference, however, lessens beyond the age of 60 years in both the sexes. From Bombay, in 1963, it was reported that the ratio of men to women getting heart attacks was as high as 12.8 to 1 for subjects under 30 years of age; for the entire series comprising all age groups, it was only 3.7 to 1. Similarly, from the USA, it has been reported that in people between 30 and 44 years of age, the male to female ratio was 13 to 1; but for the age group 45 to 62 it was 2 to 1. Furthermore, the average age of women who had heart attack was higher than that of men.

What causes more frequent occurrence of heart attacks in men? Various explanation have been offered. They relate to the environments as well as the biology associated with the male sex.

As regards the environments, it is stated that in general, the quantity of food, fats and sugar taken by men is greater than that by women. More men smoke than women. Men are more exposed to the competitive stresses of modern living.

Biologically, it has been found that normal young women have a relatively lower serum cholesterol level, lesser amount of low-density lipoproteins (LDL) and a higher concentration of high-density lipoprotein than normal young men. This sex difference disappears after the menopause.

These observations suggest that female sex hormones, the oestrogens, hinder the onset of atherosclerosis by their effect upon the quality and quantity of the fat in their blood.

The incidence and severity of coronary artery atherosclerosis in women, whose both the ovaries have been removed (because of some disease), are reported to be greater than in control females and to approximate those in men of the same age group. If, however, such women in whom the ovaries were removed, are treated with oestrogens, the incidence and severity of coronary heart disease lessens significantly. Conversely, the incidence and severity of atherosclerosis has been reported to be much less in men treated with oestrogens for carcinoma of the prostate than in control series.

Use of oestrogens, in general practice, for prevention of coronary heart disease, however, cannot be advised because of severe and unpleasant side-effects such as swelling of the breasts, impotence, nausea, vomiting, irritability, etc. and uncertainty regarding possible long term dangers.

Family History

The occurrence of heart attacks in several members of a family is a common observation. It has been found that the incidence of heart attacks is nearly four times as frequent among siblings of persons (having common ancestors) with coronary disease as among siblings of persons without it.

High blood pressure (hypertension), cerebral haemorrhage or thrombosis and diabetes appear to occur with more than average frequency in some families.

33

Genetic factors seem to be involved in predisposing some families to these diseases. However, the role of common environmental factors cannot be minimised. For example, in some families there are many members who are obese; while in some such cases, genetic factors may be involved, the role of the common habit of excessive eating among all the members, certainly contributes to this obesity.

Physical Inactivity

An increased incidence of coronary heart disease has been related to lack of physical exercise and a sedentary occupation. The societies in which economic privilege and physical inactivity go hand in hand, coronary heart disease tends to be more frequent among sedentary persons. They are also the people who tend to be obese and to eat more.

Post-mortem studies reveal that less atherosclerosis is found among those accustomed to physical exercise. These findings have been substantiated by experimental studies in animals as well.

Curiously enough, in India, coronary heart disease and consequent heart attacks have been found in almost equal frequency among manual workers as among those who are in sedentary occupations. From this it may be inferred that in a disease with multiple factor etiology, the influence of one factor can be offset by a combination of other factors.

Emotional Stress

The progressive increase in the incidence of heart attacks in more industrialised countries, especially in comparison with less industrialised countries, has suggested a causal relation between the emotional stress imposed by our modern competitive, fast-paced, industrialised society and the development of coronary heart disease.

Heart attacks have been found to be more frequent in those with great ambition, compulsive striving, extreme competitiveness, drive for recognition and preoccupation with deadlines. In a study conducted abroad among women only, it was found that heart attacks were five times more frequent in pre-menopausal women who were business or professional executives than among housewives. The higher incidence in the first group was attributed to ambition and pressure imposed by a drive for achievement in a competitive society.

Whether any particular occupations cause more emotional stress than others, is true to an extent only; it depends mainly upon the individual having that occupation.

A feeling of security and love or a lack of them, also affect the disease process. This has been demonstrated by the following experimental study.

A group of investigators was studying the effects of a diet, high in fat and cholesterol in rabbits. At the end of the stipulated period the rabbits were killed, and arteries in their bodies were examined for evidence of atherosclerosis.

The results of the study should have been rather predictable, since it was known at the time from previous studies that a diet, high in fat and cholesterol would regularly cause obvious atherosclerotic changes in the arterial systems of rabbits. But when a group of test rabbits demonstrated atherosclerotic changes which were 60 per cent less than the overall group, the investigators were astonished.

There was no obvious explanation for the unexpected result. Finally, an unplanned variable in the experiment was discovered. The rabbits which were affected less severely were those who were fed and cared for by one of the investigators, and who during the course of the experiment, regularly took them from their cages and petted, stroked and 'talked' to them.

Was this mere coincidence? Many bioscientists should have considered laughable the possibility that such rabbit-human interchanges, could play a role in atherosclerotic vascular disease.

In order to test this 'coincidence', systematic controlled studies were designed in which two groups of rabbits were again fed the same diet and were treated identically except that one group was removed from their cages several times a day for petting, and were 'talked' to each time by the same person. The result? The petted and 'talked to' group once again demonstrated a 60 per cent lower incidence of atherosclerosis.

Not content with the possibility of two coincidences, the investigators repeated the study. The results were the same. In an unexplained way, the human factor emerged. Touching, petting, handing and gentle talking emerged as a crucial determinant in the disease process of atherosclerosis.

Gout and Uric Acid

The food we eat, after digestion and absorption, is metabolised to provide energy to the body for performing various functions. As a result of metabolism of food, some waste products result, one of which is uric acid. If, through an imbalance in the system, excess uric acid gets accumulated in the body, the symptoms of gout occur. In gouty patients, coronary arteries are more likely to become atherosclerosed. This was the finding of the Framingham study in the USA.

Built of the body

Some of the Western studies have indicated that body build with predominant maleness, masculinity and compactness is more liable to heart attack.

More recent studies in our country, however, do not support this view. Here a majority of heart attacks occur in people having an average build; even people with thin build are not immune to it.

Could you be a Diabetic?

		Yes	No
1.	History of diabetes in the family?	☐	☐
2.	Are you over 40-years-old?	☐	☐
3.	Are you over-weight?	☐	☐
4.	Do you eat more than people of your age?	☐	☐
5.	Do you feel thirsty more than other people?	☐	☐
6.	Do you pass urine more frequently?	☐	☐
7.	Do you feel run down and tired easily?	☐	☐
8.	Do you get boils or sores on your body?	☐	☐
9.	Do wounds take longer in you to heal?	☐	☐
10.	Have you changed glasses more frequently?	☐	☐
11.	Any loss of weight lately?	☐	☐
12.	Women: Were your babies over-weight at birth?	☐	☐
13.	Women: Do you have vaginal itching?	☐	☐

Score 1 for every 'Yes' and 0 for 'No'.

The higher your score the greater of your chances of having diabetes.

Are you Under Stress?

Life Stresses*	Mark Value
1. Death of spouse	100
2. Divorce	73
3. Marital separation from mate	65
4. Detention in jail or other institution	63
5. Death of a close family member	63
6. Major personal injury or illness	53
7. Marriage	50
8. Being fired at work	47
9. Marital reconciliation with mate	45
10. Retirement from work	45
11. Major change in health or behaviour of a family member	44
12. Pregnancy	40
13. Sexual difficulties	39
14. Gaining a new family member (e.g. through birth, adoption, or oldster moving in, etc.)	39
15. Major personal readjustment (e.g. merger, reorganisation, bankruptcy, etc.)	39
16. Major change in financial state (e.g. a lot worse off or lot better off than usual)	38
17. Death of a close friend	37
18. Changing to a different line of work	36
19. Major change in the number of arguments with spouse (e.g. either a lot more or a lot less than usual regarding child-rearing, personal habits, etc.)	35
20. Taking on a mortgage greater than Rs. 80,000 (e.g. purchasing a home, business , etc.)	31
21. Foreclosure on a mortgage or loan	30
22. Major change in responsibilities at work (e.g. promotion, demotion, lateral transfer)	29
23. Son or daughter leaving home (e.g. marriage, attending college, etc.)	29
24. In-law troubles	29
25. Outstanding personal achievement	28

*Holmes T.H. and R.H. Rahe, "The Social Readjustment Rating Scale", *Journal of Psychosomatic Research* II (1967); 213.

Life Stresses*	Mark Value
26. Wife beginning or ceasing work outside the home	26
27. Beginning or ceasing formal schooling	26
28. Major change in living conditions (e.g. building a new home, remodelling, deterioration of home or neighbourhood)	25
29. Revision of personal habits (dress, manners, association, etc.)	24
30. Troubles with the boss	23
31. Major change in working hours or conditions	20
32. Change in residence	20
33. Changing to a new school	20
34. Major change in usual type and/or amount of recreation.	19
35. Major change in church activities (e.g. a lot more or a lot less than usual).	19
36. Major change in social activities (e.g. clubs, dancing, movies, visiting, etc.)	18
37. Taking on a mortgage or loan less than Rs. 100,000 (e.g. purchasing a car, TV, freezer, etc.)	17
38. Major change in sleeping habits (a lot more or lot less sleep or change in part of day when asleep).	16
39. Major change in number of family get-togethers (e.g. a lot more or a lot less than usual).	15
40. Major change in eating habits (a lot more or a lot less food intake or very different meal hours or surroundings).	13
41. Vacation	12
42. Christmas	13
43. Minor violation of the law (e.g. traffic tickets, jaywalking, disturbing the peace, etc.).	11

Interpretation

Low stress	:	0-149
Mild stress	:	150-199
Moderate stress	:	200-299
Major stress	:	300 or more

Heart Attack Risk Calculator

Score	0	1	2	3
Predisposing Factors				
1. Family history of heart attack	Nil	Parents/siblings after age 60	Parents/siblings before age 60	Parents/siblings/uncles/aunts before age 60
2. Sex	Female before menopause	Male/or post-menopause female	Male/or post-menopause female	Male/or post-menopause female
3. Age	10-40	41-50	51-60	Over 60
4. Blood pressure: Systolic Diastolic	Under 120 Under 89	120-139 90-99	140-159 100-119	160-over 120-over
5. Diabetes	No	Yes	Yes	Yes

6.	Cigarette smoking	No	Up to 10 cigarettes/day	Up to 20 cigarettes/day	More than 20 cigarettes/day
7.	Blood cholesterol (mg/100 ml)	Under 170	170-249	250-299	300-over
8.	Body weight	Less than normal or normal weight	Up to 5 kg over-weight	Up to 10 kg over-weight	Over 10 kg over-weight
9.	Exercise/job	Active exercise/ Active job	Nil/sedentary	Nil/sedentary	Nil/sedentary

Score	Risk
Under 5	Very low
1-10	Low
11-15	Moderate
16-20	High
Over 20	Very high.

4

Atherosclerosis : Narrowing of the Coronary Arteries

N arrowing of the coronary arteries is caused by a process called atherosclerosis. In it the inner lining of the medium-sized and large arteries becomes raised, yellow, or has pearly white streaks or plaques. This appearance is due to an irregular deposition of a soft yellow and pultaceous, fatty material, large percentage of which is cholesterol. The word atherosclerosis is derived from the Greek words *athere* meaning mush or porridge and *sclerosis* meaning hardening, which is a consequent process.

Atheromatous Plaque

The atheromatous plaque is the fundamental lesion of atherosclerosis. Plaques white to whitish-yellow in appearance, protrude into the lumen of artery. They vary in size from 0.3 to 1.5 cm in diameter, but they sometime coalesce to form larger masses. The luminal surface tends to be firm and white and deep down it is soft and yellowish.

The distribution of atherosclerotic plaques in humans tends to be quite constant and differs from the distribution of fatty streaks. The abdominal aorta is much more involved than the thoracic aorta, and aortic lesions tend to be much more prominent around the opening of its major branches. In descending order (after the lower abdominal aorta), the most heavily involved vessels are the coronary arteries (usually within the first 6 cm), the descending thoracic aorta, and the vessels of the Circle of Willis in the brain.

Fully developed atheromatous plaques may undergo a series of changes that result in so-called "complicated plaques"

1. Almost always, atheromas in advanced disease undergo patchy or massive calcification. In severe atherosclerotic disease, arteries may be converted to virtual pipe stems, and the aorta may assume an egg-shell brittleness.

2. Ulceration of the luminal surface and rupture of the atheromatous plaques may result in discharge of the debris into the bloodstream, producing microemboli.

3. Superimposed thrombosis, the most feared complication, may occur on fissured or more often ulcerated lesions. Thrombi may either occlude the lumen or become incorporated within the plaque.

4. Bleeding (haemorrhage) into the plaque may occur, especially into the coronary arteries, from rupture of either the lining membrane or the thin-walled capillaries that supply blood to the plaque. The resulting collection of blood (hematoma) may remain localized within the lining membrane or rupture into the lumen.

5. Although atherosclerosis is basically an intimal disease, i.e. of the lining membrane of the blood vessels, in severe cases the underlying vessel wall undergoes considerable pressure, atrophy and loss of elastic tissue, causing sufficient weakness to permit aneurysmal dilatation.

While atherosclerosis is a universal disease, "complicated lesions" are seen only in individuals with extremely advanced disease.

While any form of atheromatosis is serious, it is the "complicated lesion", in particular superimposed thrombosis that gives the disease its grave clinical significance.

Pathogenesis of Atherosclerosis

Any concept of pathogenesis of atherosclerosis should take into consideration some well-established observations:

1. It must explain some of the important epidemiologic and geographic findings, in particular, the increase in severity with age,

the sex difference, the striking geographic and national differences, the great variation in severity among individuals of comparable age, and the role of the major risk factors;

2. It must account for the presence of cholesterol within the atheromatous lesions and the manner by which hyperlipidemia predisposes to atherosclerosis.

No single theory copes adequately with these observations. The first theory termed the "imbibation hypothesis" proposed by Virchow in 1856, held that a principal factor in progression of the plaque is increased passage from the arterial lumen and accumulation in the arterial intima of plasma constituents (mainly fat). The second or "encrustation theory", often ascribed to Rokitansky, postulated that small thrombi composed of platelets, fibrin and leucocytes—all constituents of the blood collected over the areas of injury of the blood vessel lining, and the organization of such thrombi and their gradual growth resulted in plaque formation.

Modern theory incorporates both the earlier theories: it states that the lesions of atherosclerosis are initiated as a response to some form of injury to arterial lining (endothelium). Focal sites of injury lead to increased permeability to plasma constituents such as lipoproteins and permit platelets to adhere to the subendothelial tissue, aggregate and release the contents of their granules.

Some aspects of lipid metabolism that are particularly relevant to this disease are as follows:

1. Full-blown atherosclerosis can be produced in almost all species of experimental animals by feeding them diets that raise the plasma cholesterol level.

2. Symptomatic atherosclerosis develops infrequently in man, even in the face of other predisposing factors unless the mean plasma cholesterol exceeds 160 mg/100 ml.

3. The probability of the development of myocardial infarction increases in proportion to the plasma cholesterol level.

4. Genetically determined disorders that cause elevated plasma or tissue cholesterol levels, such as familial hypercholesrolemia, produce fatal atherosclerosis in childhood despite the lack of any other contributing factors such as hypertension, smoking or diabetes

mellitus.

5. Although trauma to the arterial lining causes thickening of the arterial wall in experimental animals, the resultant lesion either regresses or resembles a benign scar unless the animal's cholesterol level is elevated, at which time lipid is deposited in the lesion and life-threatening atherosclerosis results.

6. The lipid in atheromatous plaques is largely derived from the lipoproteins in the bloodstream.

In coronary arteries, atherosclerotic lesions are most prominent in the main stems, the highest incidence being a short distance beyond the aortic opening. Atherosolerosis is nearly always found in the portions of the vessels which are not embedded inside the heart muscle. The degree to which the lumen is narrowed varies, but once the process is present, the whole lining of the vessel is usually involved. A single tiny plaque occluding an otherwise normal coronary artery is rare.

Researches by William L. Proudfit and his colleagues at the Cleaveland Clinic, Ohio, USA, found that advanced coronary disease has poorer prognosis than mild disease. Lesions of single arteries are associated with high survival for four years, after which the survival curve falls more rapidly, probably due to development of multi-vessel disease. The prognosis is much worse for disease of three major branches or the left main artery.

5

Coronary Thrombosis and Myocardial Infarction

C oronary arteries that have suffered progressive atherosclerosis and narrowing over long decades are liable to become blocked. In a series of 6,800 consecutive post-mortems, coronary blockage was superimposed on atherosclerosis in about 92 per cent of the cases. Of these, 43 per cent were due to thrombosis, 41 per cent to progressive atherosclerotic narrowing until the artery was completely blocked, and 8 per cent to bleeding into the wall of the vessels leading to blockage of lumen.

Coronary Thrombosis

In the third stage of atherosclerosis, complications develop over the atheromatous plaques, one of them being formation of an ulcer. Such an ulcer and discontinuity of the inner lining of the blood vessel attracts to it blood platelets (thrombocytes), which adhere together and at the site of the ulcer, a collection of them forms a thrombus, which occupies a space in the lumen of the blood vessel and may completely block it in the process of trying to seal the ulcer. Collection and stickiness of the platelets is known to be enhanced in persons who have a raised level of cholesterol in the blood and particularly after a heavy fatty meal.

In post-mortem examination of the hearts in persons who died of heart attacks, it was found that more than one thrombi form in the coronaries and the fresh and the old coronary blockades are usually found in the same heart. Fresh thrombi appear red and are soft and friable. They are loosely adherent to the arterial wall and can be easily dislodged. The old thrombi appear brownish and more firmly attached.

Eventually fibrosis appears in the thrombus and the pigment disappears from it. The thrombus now becomes firm and gray and is securely attached to the wall of the artery. Recanalisation of the lumen occurs commonly and may lead to a partial but inadequate re-establishment of the circulation. Often it is impossible to determine whether we are dealing with an old recanalised thrombotic blockage or with extreme atherosclerotic narrowing or obliteration of the lumen.

Cardiac Infarction: Death of the Heart Muscle

Thrombus formation and complete blockage of the coronary artery allows no blood to pass through it to supply oxygen to that part of the heart muscle. The result is a severe injury, destruction and death of that part of the heart muscle. The process is called Infarction of Cardiac Infarction (*cardia* means heart).

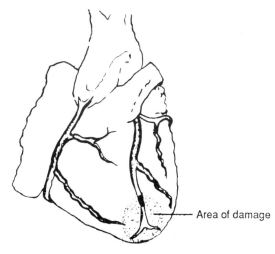

Area of damage

Fig. 7   Thrombosis and Infarction

The location and extent of the infarct depend upon many factors. These include the size and location of nearby blood vessels, the degree of narrowing of unblocked vessels, the volume of the collateral circulation in vessels, etc. Let us consider these factors one by one.

Areas of Infarctions

Artery	Area
Left anterior descending coronary artery (40 to 50%)	Anterior wall of the left ventricle near apex; anterior two-thirds of intraventricular septum.
Right coronary artery (30 to 40%)	Posterior wall of the left ventricle; posterior one-third of the interventricular septum.
Left circumflex coronary artery (15 to 20%)	Lateral wall of left ventricle

Blockage of any one of the major coronary arteries is usually followed by a cardiac infarct; blockage of any of the smaller branches rarely causes significant cardiac damage.

The frequency of the arterial involvements and the resultant areas of infarction are as follows:

The probability of cardiac infarction increases, the nearer of the site of blockage is to the origin of a major coronary artery. The more distant the blockage, the more vessels are available proximal to be blockage to provide a collateral circulation.

Sudden complete blockage in a normal large coronary artery is almost always followed by an infarct because an adequate collateral circulation has not been established. With progressive narrowing before blockage, as happens in coronary atherosclerosis, a gradual progressive increase in the relative blood flow through collateral vessels develops. In such a case, when complete obstruction occurs, the part of the heart muscle affected may be receiving its major supply from these enlarged collateral vessels, and the blockage of the original supplying vessel may not be of serious consequence.

Cardiac infarction is less likely to follow coronary blockage if the other major vessels are normal than if one of the other are already blocked or extremely narrowed. Under the latter circumstances, the possibility that the remaining vessels will provide an adequate collateral circulation is less than if they were normal. In fact, the first coronary artery blockage often causes no infarction because an adjacent major artery or a more proximal branch of the same artery provides sufficient blood to the affected area. This blockage may, however, result in less supply of oxygen (anoxia) being supplied to the heart muscle when the work of the heart is increased, and may be manifested clinically by anginal pain on physical exertion. If the second major artery which provided the collateral circulation is then occluded, a cardiac infarct usually results because the first major artery supplying the area of the heart muscle is already closed.

The extent of the infarct varies considerably from a small patch 1 to 2 cm. in diameter to widespread areas which extend through and through from the inside to the outside of the heart.

Cardiac infarction is confined almost exclusively to some portion of the left ventricle or the interventricle septum. The right ventricle is involved rarely.

Appearance of an Infarct

Myocardial infarcts less than 6 to 12 hours old, are usually inapparent on gross examination. A slight pallor may be present.

By 18 to 24 hours, the infarct is usually more clearly anaemic and grey-brown, contrasting with the surrounding normal red-brown myocardium. The consistency is still unaltered.

Between the second and fourth days, the necrotic focus becomes more sharply defined with a hyperemic border. The central portion is distinctly yellow-brown and soft.

Between the fourth and tenth days, the infarct is easily distinguished and varies from yellow-grey to bright yellow. The central necrotic tissue is maximally soft and often contains areas of bleeding (haemorrhage). The margins are intensely red and highly vascularized.

Becoming grossly apparent on approximately the tenth day,

there is progressive replacement of the necrotic muscle by the ingrowth of fibrous, vascularized scar tissue. In most instances, the scarring is well advanced by the end of the sixth week, but the time required for total replacement depends upon the size of the original infarct.

6

Diagnosis of Heart Attack

H eart attacks do not respect time, place or circumstances. These can happen to anyone, anytime, and apparently out of the blue, perhaps even depriving the unsuspecting victim of life.

Pain

The first symptom of heart attack, in a majority of the cases, is a severe and prolonged pain in the middle of the front of the chest. In some, the pain may be severe enough to be described as the worst pain the patient has ever experienced. The pain is often accompanied by weakness, sweating, nausea, vomiting, giddiness and anxiety.

The patient may be stricken while at rest or at work, awake or asleep. Master and his colleagues in 1941 noted that among 1108 heart attacks, 52 per cent occurred while the patient was asleep or resting, 21 per cent during mild routine activity, 16 per cent while the patient was walking and 9 per cent during moderate activity. In only 2 per cent was there a history to unusual physical exertion. These figures roughly correspond to the percentage of time spent on these activities during the 24 hours.

The pain, to begin with, may be relatively mild but with persistent discomfort which soon becomes severe; or it may be terribly severe from the very start. The pain of heart attack is different from other acute pains in the chest which one might have experienced. It has the quality of constriction. To describe it, the patient uses words such as squeezing, constricting, choking, vise-like or like a heavy weight.

In most cases, the pain is situated behind the sternum. Often it spreads to both sides of the front chest, especially to the left and may reach down to the upper abdomen. The pain frequently goes up the shoulders and jaw and down both the arms. If and when it involves the neck, it gives a sensation as if some unseen hand is clutching or choking the neck.

The pain in the upper extremities, more often in the left, may either extend continuously from the shoulder to the fingers or reach only to the arm or skip directly to the forearms or wrists. There may be only a dull ache, weakness of the wrists associated with severe pain behind the sternum or a little to the left.

The pain persists in varying degree for at least an hour, but often several hours, and occasionally for one to three days. The pain may not be constant even though prolonged; after an hour or two of severe pain, it may lessen perceptibly or subside entirely only to recur for hours in irregular fashion.

If it occurs in a patient of angina pectoris, he at once realises that this is a new and different pain which began while he was sleeping or was at rest, and did not subside while he rested and also was not relieved by taking the usual dose of nitroglycerin.

The pain in heart attack is due to diminished supply of oxygen to the heart muscle and this pain is a prolonged one because obstruction somewhere in the coronary arteries has blocked the supply of blood to the affected area.

Although pain is the most common presenting symptom, it is by no means always present; a minimum of 15 to 20 per cent of myocardial infarcts are painless. The frequency of such silent infarcts is probably even higher than this estimate, because patients without pain may not seek medical attention. The incidence of painless infarcts is greater in patients with diabetes mellitus, and it increases with age. In the elderly, myocardial infarction may persent as sudden onset of breathlessness, which may progress to pulmonary oedema. Other less common presentations in the absence of pain include sudden loss of confusional state, a sensation of profound weakness, the appearance of an arrhythmia, or merely an unexplained drop in arterial blood pressure.

Shock

While pain is the most prominent symptom in most of the cases of heart attack, there are cases in which this is not so. The first and the most prominent symptom may be a state of shock in which the patient at once passes. He suddenly experiences weakness which slowly or rapidly may develop into intense prostration or collapse. He may unexpectedly slump if he is standing or walking. He may lose consciousness because of less blood going to the brain.

In milder cases, the patient may complain only of feeling weak, dizzy, faint or nauseated, or less specifically of feeling 'sick'. These symptoms may be very transient and associated with cold sweat. Sometimes there is a terrifying inexplicable fear of impending doom, out of proportion to the symptoms.

In a case of severe shock, the patient may have cold, clammy limbs and tip of the nose; a rapid, and barely perceptible pulse; pallor or bluish tinge (cyanosis) and a low blood pressure (below 80 mm. Hg.). Respiration may be rapid and shallow. The facial expression is often drawn and anxious. The patient's intellect may be clear, but often he is mentally befogged and apathetic. His temperature may be subnormal. There is notable dimunution in passing urine.

This may last from a few hours to one to four days. In fatal cases, it may persist longer and until the patient succumbs. Often in such cases, shock is accompanied by pulmonary oedema.

The symptoms of shock are due to the sharp and sudden reduction in the output of blood by the heart (cardiac output) resulting from heart injury. The term 'heart failure' does not mean that the heart has stopped working or is in danger of doing so. It only means that the heart muscle has weakened to such an extent that it is not able to pump and supply blood adequately where it is needed.

Pulmonary Oedema

A sudden onset of pulmonary oedema may be the first and is often the dominant manifestation of heart attack. Pulmonary oedema

53

is the sudden out-pouring of blood serum into the lung alveoli from the lung capillaries whose walls become more permeable because of lack of oxygen. The attack may appear suddenly and without warning, causing oppression in the chest and intense suffocating breathlessness. The respiration becomes noisy and asthmatic or bubbling in character. A copious white or pinkish foamy phlegm may be coughed up or merely wells up from the respiratory passages and out of the mouth and nasal passages. Moist rales (sounds) are heard throughout the chest in the front as well as the back. The patient may be deeply blue (cyanotic) or may present a pale appearance due to the combination of pulmonary oedema with shock.

Atypical Symptoms

A patient may complain of a strange sense of mid-sternal uneasiness associated with apprehension, and a fast pulse. If he has had a heart attack before and develops such a sensation at some later time, he must get himself examined by his doctor. Similarly, those with a family history of heart attack and those with high level of cholesterol in the blood, must get themselves examined in such a situation.

Pain or numbness in the jaw often occurs as part of radiating chest pain, but may occur alone. It usually occurs in the lower jaw, on either or both sides. Toothache may indeed be a dental problem, but if the aching tooth is a healthy one, the pain may be a symptom of heart attack.

Rarely, a heart attack may present itself as numbness of the left or both the wrists.

A sudden sweating in a middle aged or old man without any obvious reason, must be looked in for heart disease.

In a case of heart attack, when the symptoms are relatively mild or the distribution of pain atypical, the diagnosis may be very difficult indeed. The following two case reports are illustrative:

1. R.S., 54 years old, complained of pain in the upper abdomen which seemed to be due to acute inflammation of the pancreas. But the laboratory tests could not confirm this. On going over the history again, it was found that the patient had similar attacks of

pain before also for the last over a year; the pain would start on exertion of the left side in the back and would then spread to the abdomen. This was relieved on resting. An E.C.G. established the diagnosis of cardiac infarction.

2. P.R., 43 years old, had for the last six months frequent attacks of pain in the front of the chest one and a half hours after taking meals. He was being treated as a case of ulcer of the stomach. However, all the laboratory investigations including X-ray of the abdomen after swallowing barium, were negative. An E.C.G. established the diagnosis of coronary heart disease.

Heart Attacks in Younger People

More and more cases of heart attacks are being observed in younger people, below the age of 40 years, both in India and abroad. Such cases occur predominantly in young males-females forming a much smaller percentage in this group than in the older age groups. According to the studies conducted in different parts of India, male to female ratio comes to 12 to 1 in this age group.

In a study from Nagpur in 1971, it was found that of the 62 patients of heart attack in younger people below the age of 45 years, occupation-wise the figures were as follows: executives or managers 4, professionals (physicians and lawyers) 4, businessmen 11, armed forces or police service 2, skilled or semi-skilled workers (mechanics and technicians) 7, offices personnel (clerks, secretaries) 13, unskilled workers (mill-hands, labourers and farmers) 15, unemployed 3, housewives 3. From the above figures, it seems hat no one group of people in a particular occupation is more liable to get heart attacks at a relatively younger age. In another study from India — curiously enough — manual workers suffered more heart attacks in the younger age compared with those having sedenatary occupations.

The time of occurrence of heart attacks is also not related particularly to any physical activity of the patient. Thus in one series of heart attacks in younger people, in 20 cases the attack occurred while the person was asleep or was resting, during mild exertion in 10 cases, moderate physical exertion in 28 cases, and heavy physical exertion in one case only.

The first symptom of the heart attack was pain in the chest in 56, sweating in 37, breathlessness in 13, vomiting in 7, sudden unconsciousness in 6, and palpitation in 3. Sudden death after a heart attack occurs more often in the younger age group patients than in the older patients.

While the symptoms of heart attack in younger persons are more or less the same as in older people, the history of a previous angina pectoris has been found to be two and a half times less common in these patients as compared with the patients in older age groups.

No significant difference in the blood cholesterol has been reported between this group and those in the older age groups, though in both of them it is higher than in the normal controls.

Of the factors which could have brought about a heart attack in these people at a comparatively younger age, heavy smoking seems to be the most important. In a study from Poona in 1973, 68 per cent of the cases were heavy smokers. The history of diabetes, high blood pressure and of being overweight was also detected more often in this age group than in the older age-groups. So was also the case with the family history of heart attacks. The presence of these predisposing factors in combination in the same person made him a more likely candidate for a heart attack at a comparative younger age.

Signs Detected by the Doctor

When the history and symptoms of the patient are suggestive of a heart attack, the doctor, when he is called, examines the patient in order to find out the tell-tale evidence of the occurrence of the attack.

In many instances the dominant feature of the patients' presentation is the reaction to the chest pain. Patients are typically anxious and restless, attempting to relieve the pain by moving about in bed squirming, stretching, belching, or even inducing vomiting. This is in contrast to the pain of angina pectoris which causes the patient to remain relatively immobile for fear of making the pain reappear. Pallor is common and is often associated with perspiration and cold extremities.

The patient may have beads of sweat on his forehead and yet his hands and feet are cold to touch. He may have a pale look and hurried and shallow breath.

Chest Examination

Examination with the help of a stethoscope may reveal some extra sounds coming from inside the chest. These sounds —moist rales—are due to collection of phlegm at the bases of the lungs. Heart sounds may not be different from the usual lubb-dup, lubb-dup, but they may sound faint and low-pitched; just at or below the left nipple, after each lubb sound, there may be a blowing murmur. Patients who had high blood pressure before, the dup sound in the upper part of the chest a little to the left of the sternum, may be a little louder or accentuated.

Pulse

The examination of the pulse may reveal no abnormality except that it is faster than usual, 100 to 110 beats per minute. It may be low in volume. It is usually regular. When an irregularity is there or when it is beating very fast, may be over 150 beats per minute, or very slow, about 30 beats per minute, it indicates damage to the area of the heart from where the pulse beat originates.

Blood Pressure

As a rule, heart attack causes a fall in the blood pressure. This fall in blood pressure is proportionately greater in patients who had high blood pressure before. It may drop down to as low as 90 of the upper limit (systolic). Lower than 70 means that the patient is in a state of shock.

In uncomplicated cases, the blood pressure begins to rise within one to three weeks; this happens usually when the patient feels well enough to move about a little and resumes the use of his muscles.

Fever

Within 24 to 48 hours of a heart attack, and sometimes even earlier (four to eight hours), there is a moderate rise in temperature of the patient. This may go up to 100°F, and in uncomplicated cases may persist up to two to six days.

All these signs are indicative of the occurrence of a heart attack in the patient. Yet the symptoms of the patient and the signs that the doctor has discovered after a physical examination, need to be confirmed, by means of different laboratory tests which also include taking an electrocardiogram of the patient.

E.C.G. in Heart Attack

Each beat of the heart is associated with an electrical impulse which passes over the heart muscle. This electrical impulse originates in the right auricle (sino-auricular node) and travels over both the auricles in a wave-like fashion to reach a place in the wall between the ventricles (auriculo-ventricular node) and then spreads over both the ventricles.

This electrical impulse is conducted throughout the body tissues to the body surface. Here it can be recorded by placing electrodes at strategic points. The record of this electrical impulse of the heart is called an Electrocardiogram (E.C.G.).

A typical E.C.G. record of a heart beat shows a sequence of waves which have been labelled P, QRS, and T. P is due to electrical activity in the upper chambers, the auricles, and QRS, and T wave due to activity in the lower chambers, the ventricles. Since the ventricles constitute the major muscle mass, they are correspondingly responsible for the major and more important share of the final electrocardiogram. In taking an E.C.G., metallic electrodes are placed on the strategic points, i.e. the forearms, legs and over the chest of the patient. The electrodes with their connections act as leads to convey the electrical impulses of the heart from skin to the electrocardiograph, the machine. The electrodes on the limbs and the chest, convey the electrical impulse of the heart as it presents itself there. Inference based upon impulses taken at different places represents a comprehensive picture of the state of the health of the heart.

In case of injury to the heart muscle, as happens in a heart attack, the configuration of the waves, particularly of the QRS and T waves which represent the ventricles and which are often damaged in a heart attack, are changed. This is due both to the absence and/

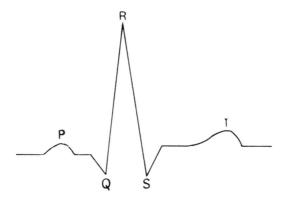

Fig. 8   ECG Wave

or diminished blood supply to the muscle fibres leading to their death or injury.

The nature of the changes in the electrical waves depends upon the site and extent of injury as well as on the time interval after which an E.C.G. has been taken after a heart attack. An E.C.G. taken immediately after a heart attack may not show any change.

The earliest changes effect the RS-T segments and are usually observed within 24 hours, rarely within a few hours, after the attack (in some instances, the RS-T changes may appear only after 2 or 3 days or even longer). The first significant abnormality is an elevation of the RS-T segment above the base line in lead I, III and a VF or in the chest leads. Characteristically, this segment presents a "high take-off" from the descending limb of the transient, lasting only a few hours or days, but it may persist for 2 to 3 weeks.

Subsequent changes produce a progressive regression of the S-T segment to the base-line and a concomitant lowering and eventual inversion of the T wave in the same lead. Simultaneously, there is often a conspicuous and sometimes broad Q wave in the same lead.

The E.C.G. changes which are regarded as characteristic of a heart attack are observed only when the infarct is large and extends the major thickness of the left ventricle.

There are innumerable wave patterns which appear in an E.C.G. after a heart attack. Only a competent heart specialist is in a position to draw inference from them, and even to differentiate an abnormal from a normal one.

Usually E.C.G. discloses changes in the impulse patterns of the heart which are not only indicative of the disease but also tell the area involved in the process. In some cases, for various reasons, an E.C.G. may not do so. This may happen:

1. When the patient has had attacks before and the picture of the previous one superimposed upon the fresh one, changes it drastically or even neutralises it.

2. The area of the heart involved in the process is too small to influence the main QRS complex and only S-T segment or T wave changes are observed.

3. Infarcts at some situations, e.g. the lateral wall, either because of the small size or because of their peculiar situation with respect to the placement of electrodes, fail to influence the recorded impulse in the E.C.G.

4. Any previous abnormality of the heart, not due to a previous heart attack, obscures the electrocardiographic pattern of a heart attack.

5. When alongwith a heart attack, some complication such as inflammation of the covering of the heart (pericarditis) occurs, so that E.C.G. changes are dominated by and are diagnostic of the pericarditis only.

6. The number of E.C.G. taken is insufficient, or the time at which these are taken in relation to the occurrence of the infarct, is not adequate to disclose the change.

7. Previous treatment by digitalis for an already existing heart disease, conceals changes due to heart attack.

8. If the chest is deformed due to any previous disease, the E.C.G. does not indicate changes due to heart attack.

An electrocardiogram is only a help in arriving at the diagnosis. It can, by no means, replace a careful history taking and physical examination of the patient. E.C.G. taken at frequent intervals and the evolving pattern of changes observed, are helpful in proper assessment of the recovery. A single E.C.G. may mislead; and E.C.G. read without knowing the history of the patient, quiet often, is misleading.

In general, if the symptoms and signs of heart attack in a patient are decidedly characteristic, there is less need for characteristic E.C.G. changes to establish the diagnosis.

Long after a heart attack has healed, an E.C.G. may continue to show changes due to the occurrence of the heart attack; these changes, however, are not as conclusive or striking as they are soon after the heart attack.

An E.C.G. in cases of through and through heart infarct returns to normal in about 10 per cent of cases, usually within a year after the attack. In the remainder, Q waves, inverted T waves or T waves of low voltage or slurred, notched and prolonged QRS complexes, persist without necessarily denoting an unfavourable prognosis.

There are other laboratory investigations, besides an E.C.G., which help in arriving at the diagnosis and in assessing the severity of the condition. Some of them are as follows:

Increase of White Blood cells (Leucocytosis)

In a normal average person, the total number of leucocytes in the blood are about 5,000 to 7,000 per c.mm. Of these 50 to 60 per cent are polymorphonuclear cells, 30 to 40 per cent lymphocytes, 3 to 4 per cent mononuclear, 3 to 4 per cent eosinophils and $^1/_2$ to 1 per cent basophils.

In a case of heart attack, the total number of leucocytes as well as the relative percentage of poly-morphonuclears is increased depending, among other factors, on the extent of the heart involved.

An increase in the white blood cell count occurs almost invariably and early, usually within 2 hours after the onset of the attack. As a rule, the white blood count varies between 12,000 to 15,000 and polymorphonuclears increase up to 75 to 90 per cent.

This increase of white blood cells (leucocytosis) recedes after a few days and usually disappears by the end of a week. Persistence of the leucocytosis thereafter suggests a complication somewhere, more probably in the lungs.

Estimation of leucocyte count and their increase is a valuable diagnostic aid in most of the suspected cases of heart attack.

Increased Erythrocycte Sedimentation Rate (ESR or BSR)

Rate of sedimentation of the red blood cells in the plasma when unclotted blood is allowed to stand under standard test conditions is a valuable diagnostic aid in cases of heart attack. Two methods are commonly used for measuring it: the Wintrobe's and the Westergren's. The level of the erythrocytes that have settled down in the tube is measured after one hour and the measurement is read as so many mm. Normal values for the Wintrobe method are 0-9 mm. in the first hour, and for Westergren a little higher, i.e. 6 to 15 mm.

The rate of sedimentation of the red blood cells (erythrocytes, *erythro* means red, *cytes* means cells) increases following a heart attack. This is noticed on the second or third day of the attack, by which time fever and leucocytosis are already present. But whereas the fever and leucocytosis usually disappear by the end of the first week, the sedimentation rate may remain raised for several weeks.

The increased sedimentation rate is attributed to a change in the composition of plasma due to the absorption of products of the necrotic heart muscle as well as to increase in plasma fibrinogen.

Blood Enzymes

During the last three decades, it has been observed that the activity level of some enzymes rises in the blood (serum) of the patient after a heart attack and this can be used in the diagnosis of the condition. These enzymes are the Serum Glutamic Oxalacetic Transaminase (in short SGOT), Creatinine Phosphokinase (CK) and the Serum Lactic Dehydrogenase (SLDH).

It was formerly believed that this rise of enzyme activity was solely due to their liberation from the damaged or dying heart muscle which is known to contain these enzymes in greater quantity than many other tissues in the body. This assertion was based upon the finding of decrease in the level of these enzymes in the injured heart muscle. This rise, however, as we know now, is not solely due to the above factor.

The normal SGOT concentration is said to be 2 to 20 units

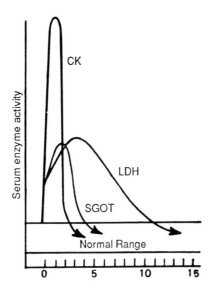

Fig. 9   Days after onset

per ml. Following a heart attack, the SGOT rises to a peak of 70 to 600 units in 12 to 48 hours, returning to normal by the fourth to seventh day. Thus, it is important to determine the SGOT activity early and to perform serial examination for proper assessment of the condition of the patient.

The enzyme SGOT is normally present in various tissues of the body, particularly in the heart muscle, skeletal muscles, kidneys, pancrease and the heart. Inflammation in any of these tissues raises the level of the SGOT in the serum. However, as a rule, it is not difficult to determine that the patient is not suffering from any of these diseases.

Enzyme creatinine phosphokinase estimation has an advantage over SGOT because the rise in its activity is more specifically related to damage to the heart.

Like the SGOT, the SLDH also shows increased activity in the serum following a heart attack. The normal total SLDH ranges between 50 and 170 units per ml. In case of heart attack, it has been found to range between 450 and 1,750 units, in one study.

Maximum levels of the SGOT and SLDH are found 24 to 48 hours after the attack. The SGOT levels usually come down to normal level by the 4th to 7th day, whereas the SLDH persists longer and comes down to normal when the patient is seen several days after the episode.

In practice, both the SLDH as well as the SGOT are determined, especially if the test is made more than 48 hours after the onset of the heart attack.

As with the SGOT, an elevated SLDH is not specific for a heart attack. It may be elevated not only in most of the conditions mentioned under the SGOT, but also as a result of some blood diseases especially as a result of destruction of red blood cells. Here also, the possibility of confusion is negligible if we take into account the history of the patient.

X-ray of the Chest

This is usually taken in a suspected case of heart attack. It may show no changes due to the attack as such, but may reveal evidence of any complication or of any other disease which the patient had before the attack, as for example, enlargement of the heart in cases in the persons who had been having high blood pressure before.

An increase in the total count of white blood cells and percentage of polymorphonuclears, raised ESR, increase in the activity of the enzymes SGOT and SLDH, coupled with a characteristic history and E.C.G. changes, clearly establishes diagnosis of heart attack.

Complications and Residual Symptoms

After a heart attack, some patients develop certain complications, which may endanger life. The commonest of them all are the irregularities in the heart beat; the other important group of complications is blocking of some arteries other than those of the heart due to embolisation. There are others also; let us take them up one by one.

Irregularities in the Heart Beat (Arrhythmias): Sudden death in a heart attack is most often due to involvement and injury of the area of the heart where the heart beat originates. When this happens, the heart either stops beating altogether or beats ineffectively—it has only a trembling movement (fibrillation).

Irregularities in the heart beat may be noticed either immediately after a heart attack or after sometime. The commonest irregularity is the insertion of extra heart beats called extrasystoles, usually arising from the ventricles, hence called ventricular extrasystoles.

Each of the heart muscle fibres is capable of beating independently. In a normal person, however, there is a controlling mechanism which makes all the fibres of the auricles or the ventricles beat at one time for an efficient functioning of heart. During a heart attack, this controlling mechanism may lose complete control over the heart beat, so that extra beats appear. If they occur too often, they interfere with effective functioning of the heart.

Other irregularities are various degrees of heart block so that there are lesser heart beats (and consequently lesser number of pulse beats per minute). This causes lesser quantity of blood being pumped by the heart to different parts of the body.

If serious irregulaties develop after a heart attack, they make an already injured heart less effective in its function, consequently making the patient more difficult to manage.

Embolism: In a healthy person, blood everywhere in the body is completely fluid, able to flow through even the minutest vessels, the capillaries. This is helped by the up and about condition of the person. A heart attack patient when he is lying down in bed, may, upon some undue pressure on the blood vessel walls in the legs, injure their inner lining so that a blood clot or thrombus forms over there. When a small piece of that clot gets detached from its original site, and flowing in the veins, through the heart and then the arteries, gets lodged in some organ, the phenomenon is called embolisation. When this happens in the lungs, it is called pulmonary embolisation (pulma means lung). It may occur while the patient is still bedridden, but frequently it develops suddenly when the patient sits up in bed, strains at stool or get out of bed for the first time.

Pulmonary embolisation usually occurs by the end of the first week, or during the second week of the onset of the heart attack. One of the first symptoms is severe pain in the chest and sometimes, spitting of blood in the phlegm. It is often difficult to distinguish between pulmonary embolisation and a fresh heart attack.

The emboli have the tendency to recur, each new embolus increasing the probability of a fatal outcome.

In a heart attack when the area involved reaches down to the inner lining of the heart (endocardium) where the blood flows, a clot may form over there, which then dislodged may go into the aorta and the arteries, going to the brain or other organs. Obstruction of a blood vessel in the brain may cause injury or death of that part, such as loss of voice, paralysis in the limbs, etc. Other emboli may lodge in the kidneys disturbing their functioning.

Here we may remember that atherosclerosis affects not only the cornoary arteries but also the arteries in the brain, kidneys and other places. Such narrowed arteries are liable to thrombus formation.

If an embolus happens to lodge in one of the main arteries of a limb, it causes excruciating pain, loss of sensation, loss of motion, absence of pulsation, blanching and coldness over the part. If it involves only a smaller limb artery, collateral circulation may come to the rescue of the part. But if it is a larger artery that is involved, gangrene of the area may occur.

Rupture of the Heart: This is one of the causes of sudden death in the first two weeks after a heart attack. One-eighth of the patients who succumb in the first three weeks after a heart attack, die from rupture of the heart.

Rupture of the heart results from a through and through laceration of an infarcted area which is still soft and necrotic.

Although high blood pressure and exertion are accessory factors favouring rupture of the heart after a heart attack, it depends primarily on the site and extent of the infarct. Rupture is also favoured by absence of a collateral and absence of fibrosis in the infarct.

Death may occur within a few minutes after the rupture, but occasionally there is a survival period of a half hour to several hours.

Rupture of the wall between the two ventricles also occurs if infarction happens to be in this area. The symptoms are those of recurrence of severe pain, breathlessness, shock and irregularities in the heart beat. The prognosis is poor; the majority of the patients dying within the first week.

Following a through and through infarct, the area of the heart involved may get fibrosed. This scarred area is weak. The pressure of blood in the heart here may cause a bulge to develop over there. This happens in roughly about 5 per cent of the cases of heart attack. X-ray and E.C.G. help to diagnose and localise the condtion. This is compatible with life, though such a diseased and weak heart may not pull the patient through for very long.

Chronic Left Ventricular Failure: If much of the heart muscle has suffered chronic malnutrition from diminished blood flowing through it, a heart attack may act as a last straw on it, under whose weight it may falter and fail. Such a patient may develop recurrent attacks of breathlessness and cough at night. These symptoms may look like those of bronchitis or asthma, but the case history of the patient, physical examination and the relevant laboratory investigations leave little doubt about the true nature of the condition.

Broncho-pneumonia: This may occur due to congestion and infection in the lungs. This is commonly a terminal or terminating event in cases that develop pulmonary oedema after a heart attack.

This is characterised by protracted or recurrent fever and chest pain clinically akin to that of pericarditis.

Most commonly it occurs in the second to the sixth week after a heart attack. The diagnosis is uaually suggested by the persistence or recurrence of chest pain. Fever is usually present. This is atrributed to an antigen-antibody response, the antigen being the heart muscle itself.

Arthritis of the Shoulder: Pain, stiffness and marked limitation of motion at the shoulder joint, shoulder girdle and arm, frequently result after a heart attack. The symptoms vary from mild pain on movement to severe pain with almost complete limitation as movement especially on lifting the arm from the side. In severe cases, the pain may persist from 6 months to 2 years.

The left shoulder and arm are usually affected, but the right side or both sides may be involved. It has been observed that it occurs less often if the patient is given greater freedom of movement after the onset of the heart attack.

Angina Pectoris: In about half the cases in which angina pectoris is absent before the attack, it develops after recovery from heart attack. If angina was present before, it persists after the attack. Only occasionally patients, who have suffered from angina, lose their pain after an attack of acute cardiac infarction; this is probably due to the fact that the heart muscle which complained as pain to oxygen lack, dies when complete block of the nourishing artery occurs.

Enlarged Heart: Heart enlargement following recovery from the heart attack is observed eventually in more than half the cases, but only as a result of associated or complicating factors, especially if there was high blood pressure before.

7

Medical Treatment of Heart Attack

A patient who has suffered a heart attack usually has severe chest pain which needs to be relieved. Besides that he may be having other symptoms like shock, pulmonary oedema, heart failure or irregularities in the beat of the heart. All this needs immediate attention.

The heart which has suffered damage is not in a position to work as effectively as before, and hence it is necessary that work load on it is reduced. This is done by providing rest and relieving apprehension and pain. Besides that, it is necessary to overcome shock and cardiac failure, if present, and to cope with dangerous irregularities of the heart or any other complication that may arise. Let us take these items one by one.

Pain

As a rule, morphine, 15 mg (but only 8 to 10 mg in an elderly) is given intramuscularly to control severe pain and any associated restlessness and anxiety at the onset of the attack. Morphine may not be given if the pain is relatively mild and can be relieved by usual analgesics. If the pain has already subsided, none of the drugs need be given however, a mild sedative may be useful. Morphine or pethidine should not be used for restlessness and anxiety in the absence of severe pain.

There is a tendency to excessive use of morphine which complicates the clinical picture and ultimately increases symptoms by further lowering the blood pressure and causing distressing nausea, vomiting, abdominal distress and depression of respiration.

Shock

Certain general measures, such as rest in bed, and alleviation of pain, restlessness and anxiety by morphine or pethidine, are indirectly helpful. The patient should lie flat in bed until an adequate blood pressure is restored, but some compromises are necessary if pulmonary oedema is also present when the patient feels better by sitting up in bed. In cold weather, body heat may be conserved by means of blankets.

Oxygen is administered continuously.

If the blood pressure has fallen very low, such drugs are given as bolster to sharply reduced quantity of blood pumped to different parts of the body (cardiac output) which is primarily responsible for low blood pressure and shock. The following drugs are intended to enable the patient to survive critical period until the heart recovers its ability to maintain the blood pressure without outside assistance.

A number of such drugs are avilable, which include levarterenal (Lovophed, Noradrenaline), metaraminal (Aramine), mephentermine (Wyamine), methoxamine (Vasoxyl) and phenylephrine (Neo-Synephrine). Angiotensin (Hypertension) has also been similarly employed. Levarterenal and metaraminal are now employed most commonly, and administered by continuous intravenous infusion. But metaraminal (Aramine) and mephentermine (Wyamine) are also often used initially by intramuscular injection to maintain blood pressure until a continuous intravenous infusion can be started.

Shock and Pulmonary Oedema

Shock and pulmonary oedema occur sometimes together and pose a difficult problem for treatment. The shock can be treated as discussed above, but due regard has to be paid to minimising the quantity of intravenous fluids injected, otherwise, it aggravates pulmonary oedema.

Control of Irregular Heart

An already damaged heart becomes more inefficient if there is superadded irregularity of the heart beat, because then it cannot pump out the blood. In such cases, control of heart rhythm by a drug or by means of an artificial pace-making device is a life-saving measure.

Artificial Cardiac Pace-makers

Heart block may occur as a manifestation of heart attack. Atrial electrical impulse fails to reach and stimulate the ventricle. The ventricles beat independently at a low rate of 25 to 50 per minute. The dangers of this situation are:

1. The slow-rate impairs cardiac output and may lead to heart failure.

2. A sudden slowing or cessation of the beat may produce syncope or death.

Although the ventricular rate can sometimes be increased by drugs such as ephedrine, iso-prenaline and the like, yet the response to drugs become less with continued use.

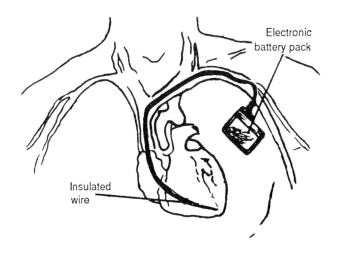

Fig. 10   Artificial Cardiac Pace-maker

Artificial electrical pace-makers have been designed to stimulate the heart at any desired rate. These can be **wholly external** using electrodes applied to the surface of the chest; **wholly internal** with a small implantable battery-operated pace-makers, which is buried in the abdominal wall and connected to the myocardial surface by wire electrodes, or combined internal and external. In the latter, the apparatus is external and the heart is stimulated either by a catheter electrode passed through the external jugular vein into the right ventricle, or by wire electrodes attached to the surface of the ventricle.

The most common form of direct cardiac pacing is the endocardial in which an electrode catheter is placed, generally in the right ventricle, through the venous route; it is employed with an external power supply for temporary pacing, or one that is implanted subcutaneously for permanent pacing. Endocardial pacing of the atrium is more difficult to achieve on a long-term basis because of electrode instability but can sometimes be achieved with placement of the pace-maker within the coronary sinus. Epicardial pacing may be carried out by suturing wire leads to the atrial or ventricular myocardium at the time of thoracotomy or by application of sutureless electrodes which screw into the myocardium. For permanent direct pacing the power supply is totally implanted.

Complete AV block in association with acute myocardial infarction occurs in less than 10 per cent of patients. The survival rate among hospitalized patients with infarction complicated by complete heart block approximates 50 per cent. The poor outlook is a reflection not only of sequelae of AV block but also of the frequently associated extensive underlying infarction. Implementation of temporary transvenous pacing reduces the mortality rate and is warranted as a protection against transitory hemodynamic disturbances accompanying block. Long-term pacing has been shown to reduce the risk of sudden death during subsequent year.

Role of Mobile Coronary Care Units

Many of the deaths after a heart attack occur in the early hours of the attack. This is due either to complete stoppage of the heart beat or due to the irregularities of the heart in which the ventricles just fibrillate ineffectively without pushing out any blood.

Mobile coronary care units can prove life saving in some cases. In one study, it was estimated that the delay between the onset of symptoms and the initiation of care is reduced from an average of 8 hours to only 1 hour 40 minutes by the help of such units.

Role of Intensive Coronary Care Units

Since mortality from arrhythmia is greatest during the first few hours after infarction, it is obvious that the effectiveness of coronary care unit relates directly to the speed with which patients come under medical observation.

The biggest delay usually is not transportation to the hospital but rather between the onset of pain and the patient's decision to call for help. This delay can be reduced by education of the public concerning the significance of chest pain and the importance of seeking early medical attention. Heart attack patients, at least those who appear more seriusly ill, should be carefully observed in an Intensive Coronary Care Unit (ICCU) during the period of greatest danger. Such units exist now in large hospitals in India.

A ICCU provides the necessary constant observation by well-trained nurses and physicians, with the aid of devices for continuous electrocardiograph monitoring, (including in some cases oscilloscopic, electrocardiographic closed-circuit television) and various recording instruments. Audiovisual alarms are activated by cardiac arrest, predetemined changes in the ventricular rate or decline in blood pressure. In particular, personnel and equipment are available constantly to apply modern methods of resuscitation for cardiac arrest including artifical ventilation, external cardiac compression and defibrillation.

Lidocaine has been identified as an anti-arrhythemic drug of unique effectiveness for the prophylactic treatment of ventricular ectopic activity in acute myocardial infarction. Ventricular fibrillation has been in many instances prevented by aggressive anti-arrhythmic drug therapy. *As a result the focus of coronary care has changed from resuscitation to prevention.*

Any substantial improvement in mortality from heart attack

depends on the reduction in deaths from the major complications of irregular heart, shock, acute pulmonary oedema and heart failure. Management of shock and heart failure demands continuous observation by skillful personnel. Control of the irregular heart offers great promise of diminishing death rate since sudden death, which occurs commonly because of ventricular fibrillation or complete stoppage of heart may be prevented by electric shock and external cardiac compression.

Devices for continuous E.C.G. monitoring have disclosed that irregularities in heart beat, sometimes of multiple variety, occur in more than 70 per cent, and serious, or potentially serious irregularities of heart such as ventricular techycardia or fibrillation or both, in 10 to 15 per cent of patients of heart attack. Prompt elimination of these irregularities may prevent the occurrence of stoppage of heart beat. Both the early recognition and treatment of these irregularities and of cardiac arrest require continuous monitoring in a specialised place with appropriate facilities, equipment and personnel.

Occasionally a question arises as to what sort of patients should be taken in ICCU and for how long should they remain there?

It has been found that about one-third to one half of deaths from heart attack occur in the first 24 hours, about 70 per cent within the first 3 days and 80 to 85 per cent in the first week. Since such a large percentage of deaths occurs within the first 5 days after a heart attack and since dangerous irregularities are likewise most frequent during this period, it is generally recommended that a 5-day stay in the ICCU should represent the usual duration, but longer stay may be desirable if indicated by the clinical course.

However, equipment alone does not ensure an effective coronary care unit. Of prime importance is the organization of a highly trained team of nurses who can recognize arrhythmias, adjust the dosage of anti-arrhythmic drugs, and perform cardiac resuscitation, including the application of electric shock when necessary. A physician should be available at all times, but many lives have been saved because nurses have treated ventricular tachycardia or fibrillation before the physician's arrival.

Sudden Stoppage of Heart and External Cardiac Compression

In some cases of heart attack, the heart stops beating suddenly before there is any opportunity to take the patient to the hospital. In such a case, give a hard blow with your fist over the heart on the chest. Sometimes, the heart starts beating at once.

If it does not do so, one has to resort to external heart compression. The method of doing it is simple but it is worthwhile only if a physician or a layman is familiar with the technique and can apply it at a moment's notice.

The principle is that by applying firm pressure over the lower half of the sternum, one can readily compress the heart, forcing blood into the aorta and pulmonary artery. Releasing this pressure produces a negative intra-thoracic pressure, causing blood to be drawn into the heart from the body veins into the right side of the heart.

To apply external cardiac compression, place the patient on a hard surface, with his legs a little raised. His neck should be extended. Place the heel of your one hand on lower half of the sternum, parallel with long axis of the body. Then place the heel of the other hand over the fist. With your arms in a vertical position, elbows straight, exert rhythmic pressure directly downward from your shoulders, using the weight of your upper body pressing directly down toward the spine. Make the downward stroke rapidly, hold it approximately half a second, and then instantly release it, giving the chest wall a chance to recoil. Repeat the whole procedure once a second or even slightly faster.

Mouth to mouth artificial respiration is also given.

There is no time to waste at all in cases of sudden cardiac arrest. Even if the patient seems not to be responding, never stop resuscitative efforts until about 15 minutes are past.

When the patient is already connected to a monitoring device, in a case of a cardiac arrest, the treatment is to give a defibrillating shock at once.

If fortunately, you are able to bring back the patient's pulse and respiration, he needs to be carefully observed and nursed for at least 72 hours.

Diet of Heart Attack Patient

In the first week, the diet must be varied according to the patient's condition. When he is severely ill, he may take only small amounts of fluid at a time, such as fruit juices, milk, broth, tea, water etc. Care should be taken to avoid distressing abdominal distension in persons intolerant to milk or excessive amounts of fruit juice. Salt (sodium chloride) intake should be restricted if there is evidence of heart failure.

When they are tolerated, soft foods are allowed in addition to fluids. Cooked cereals, and simple puddings may be given at brief intervals, but only in small amounts at any one time.

The intake of food is increased gradually as the patient is permitted to get out of bed and resume moderate activity. A lower caloric intake is to be given for those who are overweight so as to reduce in weight.

The diet should eliminate foods which are usually difficult to digest and which are likely to cause distension. Raw fruits, fruit juices in excess, fried foods and gravies, spices and condiments, fatty meats, cheese, nuts, dates, chocolates should be avoided.

Smoking should be avoided and it is better to leave the habit at this time. Alcohol—if one is used to it—may be taken in small quantity. Coffee may also be taken in moderation, if one is used to it.

After a severe attack, it is undesirable that the patient be disturbed or urged to move his bowels for the first three days, as straining at stool may be a dangerous exertion. Usually the patient is constipated during this period because of the low intake of food and specially because of the administration of morphia or pethidine. Soft easy bowel movements may be effected with the aid of liquid paraffin.

How much Bed Rest is Advisable?

Rest in bed is the first instruction given to a heart attack patient so as to lessen the work load on his heart. But for how long should he rest? A clear answer to this query was not available till lately. Earlier, most of the physicians advocated a much longer period of rest.

Nowadays, a rest period of six weeks is considered safe on the basis of the following observations:

1. Most of the deaths and complications from heart attack occur during the first week, a more moderate in the second week and relatively few in the third week. For this reason, a minimum of two to three weeks of rest is essential.

2. Experimental studies show that two or three weeks are necessary for the development of collateral circulation to supplement the interrupted blood supply.

3. About six weeks are required for the cardiac infarct to be converted into firm scar.

Keeping in view the above observations, some modifications may be made depending upon the severity of the attack and the needs of the individual.

Rest in bed does not imply complete immobilisation or even complete restriction to bed for every minute of that period. As soon as possible after the onset of the attack, the patient can be allowed to feed himself, to move freely in bed and to perform leg exercise (especially up and down movements at the ankle and knee) at regular frequent intervals. He can even be allowed the facility of sitting on the commode once a day at a regular hour. Furthermore, within the confines of his bedroom or his hospital room, he is permitted moderate liberties which do not involve more than the simplest exertion and do not result in mental or emotional strain.

Those who have experienced only small patches of infarcts with no complications, and made a rapid recovery, are often restricted to bed or inactivity for only two or three weeks, after which they are allowed to return to work. On the other hand, a further period of weeks or months of rest is necessary in some patients with complications or persistent symptoms.

The strictness with which bed rest is enforced has to be weighed judiciously in individual cases against the risk of venous thrombosis and pulmonary embolism, deterioration of morale, the frequency of constipation and abdominal distention, the circulatory strain often involved in the use of the bed pan, the occurrence of disabling aches and pain in the back or the shoulders, the development of bed sores, the occurrence of urinary disability or retention of urine in patients with prostate enlargement.

When the patient can, or when he gets breathlessness on lying down straight in bed, part of the time he can be made to sit in an arm chair.

Debilitating Effect of Long Bed Rest

Rest in bed for a duration longer than a week has by itself a debilitating effect on the general health of a person, even if he or she is a normal person. Saltin and his colleagues in 1968, demonstrated this effect clearly. They took two groups of apparently healthy college students, one group composed of physically active boys, members of the university team and the other group of a more sedentary students. These young men were put to a strict bed rest for 21 days. Both groups of students sustained a marked decrease in maximal oxygen uptake, and they took a considerable time to return to normal heart function; so much so that three weeks of training was required to restore these young men to their pre-bed maximal oxygen uptake.

After rest in bed for a few weeks, a given physical exercise or exertion increases heart rate more than before the rest period. It also decreases lung volume and the vital capacity. There is a decrease in contractile strength of the muscles, particularly noticeable in the limb muscles.

This indicates that the weakness and fatigue so often described by the heart attack patient after several weeks of bed rest, might be related more to the enforced treatment than to the underlying disease.

Lesser stress on strict prolonged bed rest in uncomplicated cases and a more active programme of rehabilitation of the patient so that he could return to his work, has been found to be useful for the following reasons:

1. The patient loses his or her unconscious anxiety,

2. He/She returns to his/her work and to better economic conditions,

3. He/She becomes more cheerful and physically healthy; and above all,

78

4. Active life provides early and better collateral circulation in place of the blocked coronary arteries so that he stands lesser chances of getting further heart attacks.

All these advantages have made cardiologists advocate and arrange more active physical exercise programmes for their patients.

In suggesting rehabilitative physical exercises to the patient who has had a heart attack, a balance is to be struck between keeping the patient physically fit and not to put any strain upon his heart. The criteria used are to see that the pulse rate of the patient does not rise more than 10-15 per minute from the resting state to that of exercise; also that his blood pressure does not rise by more than 5 points.

The choice of a particular set of exercises for an individual patient is left to the physiotherapist under whose guidance the exercises are learnt and undertaken.

After training, a patient's response to the same work load is characterised by a lesser increase in heart rate, a lesser increase in blood pressure and a lesser increase in the output of blood by the heart. Furthermore, there is a reduced tendency to get attacks of angina pectoris, and decreased or absent ST-T changes in the E.C.G.

Hospital versus Home-Care

Most patients with uncomplicated or relatively mild heart attack can be treated satisfactorily at home. However, there is a constant danger of a serious irregularity of the heart beat or other complication which is less likely to be recognised and treated early and effectively at home than in a hospital.

In general, hospitalisation is preferable, especially if the severity of the attack and its complications warrant frequent and prompt medical attention, obtained at home, when the patient's activities or intrusions by relatives, friends or business associates can only be controlled in the hospital, or when other environmental conditions at home are undesirable. The patient's progress as determined by frequent observation and by E.C.G. or other laboratory tests, can usually be followed more easily at a hospital.

The physician should not be deterred from hospitalisation of the patient because of the exaggerated fear of moving the patient, provided this can be done by ambulance with the aid of trained attendants. An injection of morphine or pethidine should be administered for pain or an intramuscular injection of 5 mg of Aramine for low blood pressure if necessary before transporting him, and oxygen therapy should be available or provided during transportation.

Sometimes hospitalisation appears preferable to home treatment for the first 2 or 3 weeks, after which treatment may be continued at home. Under these circumstances also, there is no objection to moving the patient if he is recovering satisfactorily, if no excessive exertion on his part is required in the transfer, which should be done by ambulance.

Alongwith physical rest, a complete mental rest and protection from emotional strain is necessary for a patient of heart attack. These aims can be attained by isolation of the patient from outside communications and contacts which produce mental strain or upset him emotionally, by confident reassurance that he will get well, and efficient examination and care of the patient on the part of the doctor and nurse with as infrequent disturbance as possible. About 20 to 25 per cent of the patients who have a heart attack, end up in sudden death.

Of those who are spared this catastrophe, the first 24 hours are the most crucial. Thereafter up to 10 days of the attack are still dangerous. Inclusive of the sudden deaths, up to 30 to 40 per cent heart attack patients die in this period. After that the chances of survival improve.

Prognosis after a Heart Attack

In an individual case, the following factors influence the prognosis after a heart attack.

1. The mortality increases with the increasing age of the patient.

2. The mortality is higher among the patients who have high blood pressure than in those who have normal before the attack.

3. The mortality is significantly higher in patients presenting a history or evidence of previous heart attacks.

4. Those with a history of angina pectoris have a poorer prognosis than those who never had angina before.

5. When severe pain persists for more than 24 hours, and is incompletely relieved by morphine or pethidine, the outlook for survival is usually unfavourable.

6. When a heart attack is accompanied by an extreme degree of shock, or when evidence of shock persists after several days, the outlook is unfavourable. Mortality rates between 70 and 90 per cent have been reported for patients with shock and blood pressure persistently under 80 mm Hg.

7. A temperature of 104°F or higher, or a white blood count above 20,000 denotes extensive or progressive heart involvement or a serious complication and is associated with a high mortality.

8. The mortality is strikingly higher among diabetic than among non-diabetic patients.

9. The mortality rate is significantly increased in the presence of severe types of irreggularities such as ventricular tachycardia or heart block.

10. The occurrence of emboli in the lung, brain, other organs or the extremities is associated with a high mortality.

11. Among men having heart attack for the first time, those who engage in the least physical activity before the attack, experience a mortality rate three times greater than those who are engaged in strenuous physical activity.

12. The location of the infarct in itself as shown by an E.C.G. has no prognostic significance.

After recovery from a heart attack, the prognosis of a patient is rated much more favourable now than was formerly. At least 40 per cent of the patients survive for more than 10 years, and at least 70 per cent for 5 years or longer. The duration of survival is significantly less if hypertension is associated than in its absence.

The prognosis is particularly favourable in patients who recover completely after a heart attack without subsequent angina pectoris, unusual fatigability or evidence of heart failure, diabetes, hypertension or obesity and those who do not smoke.

Chances of Subsequent Heart Attacks

Long term clinical observations show that additional attacks recur in about 30 per cent of cases, usually within two years after the first attack.

Post-mortem studies, however, reveal a much higher incidence.

Subsequent episodes are often overlooked because the clinical features either are not as characteristic as those of the first attack or are overshadowed by symptoms and signs of congestive heart failure and because the E.C.G. changes when superimposed or previous abnormalities are often not specific.

Each additional heart attack either increases the probability of a fatality or leaves the patient more subject to the development or intensification of congestive heart failure or disabling attacks of angina pectoris than after the first attack.

Rehabilitation of the Patient

Until about 1930, a patient who suffered a heart attack was considered to be totally and permanently disabled and the possibility that he might one day resume work was, therefore, never considered. This brought about more disability and neurosis in the patient.

In the 1950s it was realised that prolonged and strict bed rest is not essential. This realisation favourably influenced the course of the disease, and besides less morbidity, the mortality decreased from the expected 15 per cent to 10 per cent because of the lesser complications developing due to prolonged rest in bed.

Nowadays, after a six-week period of rest in bed, the physician wants his patient to come back to his work; of course the patient has to observe some precautions and moderation in day to day activities.

Role of Yoga in Rehabilitation

A programme of *asanas* (postures) for rehabilitation of patients after the heart attack has been suggested by yoga experts from Poona. Yogic postures are not meant to build muscles but intend to relax the body and the mind.

These postures are started only after the patient has become symptom-free, has no complication and heart rate and blood pressure are stable. In some cases, it is necessary to start with simpler postures initially and subsequently builtup. These postures are performed under the close guidance of an expert.

A total of 10 postures are selected for the purpose. These are steadily maintained for 5 to 15 seconds but without any discomfort. Movements are slow and without jerks. Patients are instructed to watch and guide their breathing normally. The same posture is repeated three times. In between two postures, the person relaxes as completely as possible.

The postures are done in the morning before breakfast. The person lies relaxed on his back. The following postures may prove useful:

1. Lie relaxed on the back. Raise arms and extend them back, parallel with the head.

2. Lie in the same position as above. Stretch both the arms at right angles to the body.

3. Lie in the same position as in No. 2. Keep arms by the side of the body.

4. Lie in the same position as in No. 2 and 3 with arms by the side of the body. Lift right leg from the hip joint to an angle between 15° to 45° and maintain it for 5 to 15 seconds and then gradually bring it down on the ground.

5. Do No. 4 with the left leg.

6. Raise both legs together.

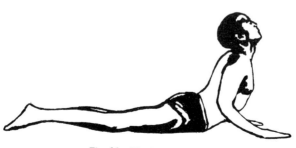

Fig. 11   Bhujanga Asana

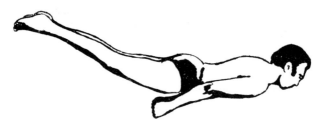

Fig. 12   Salabh Asana

7. Cobra posture (*Bhujanga asana*): Lie down on the belly in a completely relaxed state with palms beneath the corresponding shoulder. Then slowly raise the head and upper portion of the body up to the umbilicus just as a cobra raises its hood, with face looking up, supporting the body on partially extended elbows.

8. Semi-locust posture (*Ardha-salabh asana*): Lie down on your belly with hands by the side of the body, palms facing down. With right knee extended, lift the right leg back from the thigh to an angle of 15° to 45°.

9. Do No. 8 with left leg.

10. Locust posture (*Salabh asana*): Lie down as in No. 8 and No. 9. Raise both legs up after inspiration.

By performing these yogic postures, the patients felt more cheerful, reassured, unfatigued and 'returned' to their previous occupations and routine.

Whether it is by means of yogic postures or otherwise, the idea of rehabilitating a heart attack patient is to keep all parts of the body in a working condition without straining the heart so that he is in fit condition to resume his physical work.

Suggested Menu for a Heart Attack Patient

Breakfast

    Orange juice
    Skimmed milk and cornflakes
    Skimmed milk—8oz
    Toast, unbuttered—2 slice
    Tea or coffee with skimmed milk

Lunch

    Chapatti or boiled rice—2 chapattis or 4oz rice
    Boiled vegetable or boiled beans or lentil—4oz
    Skimmed milk curd *(dahi)*
    Cheese prepared from skimmed milk
    Fresh fruit

Dinner

    Tomato juice
    Green salad
    Boiled or roasted chicken, or lean meat
    Vegetable or green peas, boiled with slight addition of
    ground-nut oil
    Mashed potatoes made with ground-nut oil
    Pudding made with skimmed milk.

8

Surgical Treatment of Heart Attack

Attempts have been made to help the patients of coronary heart disease by means of surgery. The essential lesion being narrowing or obstruction of the coronary arteries, the surgical attempts have been directed the much needed blood to the heart muscle indirectly by grafting some other source of blood to it.

After the trial of many indirect and some direct techniques in experimental animals and patients, all of which either failed or succeeded only partially, in 1967, Dr. Rine Favalore, removed a section of the saphenous vein from the leg, grafted on end of it into the aorta and the other end into the coronary artery, at a place where it was healthy, thus bypassing the obstructed or narrowed segment of the coronary.

Since this procedure bypasses the coronary obstruction, it is called coronary bypass operation and since it connects the aorta directly with the coronary artery, it is called aorto-coronary procedure.

Bypass Operation Technique

A combined surgical procedure now undertaken is as follows. The patient is put to sleep with a general anaesthetic. An incision is made in a leg to remove a segment of saphenous vein from groin to knee, which is then tested for its patency and all clear calibre.

Another surgeon opens up the chest at the same time. The patient is connected to the heart-lung machine. This consists of a pump and an oxygenator. Blood is withdrawn from the vena cavae, passed through the oxygenator and returned into the arterial circulation through the femoral artery or ascending aorta. The blood is thus diverted completely from the heart and lungs (extracorporeal), but a good supply of well-oxygenated blood is made available to the vital organs. Heart-lung machines provide the surgeon with enough time for intracardiac surgery of between two or three hours with safety.

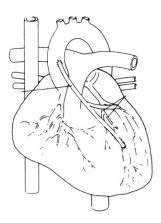

Fig. 13   Bypass Operation

This operation is done on the patient when the temperature of his body is less than normal (hypothermia) around 29° to 30° C. This reduces the oxygen requirements of the vital organs and thus the operative procedure can be carried along for a longer time.

The surgeon touches two electrodes to the heart and passes in a shock. The heart begins to fibrillate, i.e. instead of contracting as usual, it begins to quiver only, so that it can be handled. Now the surgeon cuts away the overlying tissues, and comes to the coronary artery which is blocked. A clamp is put on the aorta which cuts off the flow of blood to the coronary arteries and the heart stops making any movement. During this period, the surgeon takes a section of the vein, cuts the end obliquely, and with suture material as fine as a thin hair, stitches it to a slit in the aorta. The other end of the vein is stitched on the coronary artery beyond the obstruction or narrowing. This procedure is then repeated for any other coronary vessel where bypass is necessary.

After this is done, the heart is restarted and the patient is disconnected from the heart-lung machine. Improvement is evident at once. Through the bypass, more blood flows to feed the heart muscle.

Surgical techniques have been developed to the point where up to bypass can be fixed in one single patient and myocardial revascularization can be safely performed even in case with markedly impaired myocardial function.

Indications for Surgery

Most patients who have coronary artery narrowing and are symptomatic in the form of having angina pectoris or having had a heart attack, can be managed fairly well with drugs and need no surgical intervention. The decision, whether bypass surgery is indicated depends, besides other factors, on:

1. How old the patient is?
2. How able is he to work or live the kind of life he desires?
3. How incapacitating is the angina?
4. Are symptoms progressive?
5. How well does he respond to medicines?
6. What are the results of the exercise test?
7. What is the severity of coronary narrowing?

In addition to the above, the doctor and the patient have to weigh the potential benefits of the operation against the risks of surgery.

A pre-requisite to coronary bypass surgery is knowing the state of health or disease of the coronary arteries. This can be found out by a procedure called coronary arteriography.

Coronary Arteriography

Coronary arteriography is the only method which can provide

unequivocal diagnostic information concerning the presence or absence of coronary atherosclerosis in living patients. It also permits estimation of the severity of obstructive lesions which may be present.

This involve the injection of a special dye into the coronary arteries. The dye can be seen on X-ray film as it flows through the arteries and thus any obstruction in the coronary arteries can be seen and the location and severity of narrowing can be pinpointed.

An area of the groin or arm is numbed with local anaesthetic (such as novocaine). One of the blood vessels passing through the arm or groin is entered by a needle or tiny incision, and a thin, long tube (a catheter) is passed through this vessel to an area just outside the heart, where its tip is directed into the opening of the coronary arteries. Then the dye is injected into the arteries. X-ray movies or still shots are taken and the films are analyzed to locate regions of narrowing within the cronary arteries.

Opinion is nearly unanimous that coronary arteriography is indicated in the following specific situations:

1. Patients with either chronic, stable angina pectoris, or unstable angina, who are refractory to medical treatment, and others who on clinical grounds are considered to be candidates for coronary bypass surgery.

2. Patients with a variety of diagnostic problems in which diagnosis of coronary artery disease leading to diminished blood supply to the heart muscle, needs to be established or ruled out. Six groups of patients exemplify the latter situation (Brunwald and Cohn, 1983):

a. Patients with negative exercise tests and a disabling chest pain syndrome. Included in this group are patients with a chest pain but who need unequivocal evidence either for psychological reasons or for personal decisions relating to career-planning, family planning, insurability, etc.

b Patients with frequent hospital admissions with the diagnosis of possible myocardial infarction which had never been substantiated and in which the diagnosis of coronary atherosclerosis has not been established.

c. Commercial and military flight personnel or others with careers in which more than individual safety is concerned and in whom there is a reasonable doubt as to the status of the coronary circulation.

d. Patients with severe aortic valve disease and angina pectoris in whom this symptom could be secondary of the valvular lesions and/or to coronary arteriosclerosis.

e. Young patients (under age 45) with angina or documented myocardial infarction in whom none of the risk factors associated with premature coronary disease can be identified and who may not have extensive coronary atherosclerosis, and, hence, a more favourable prognosis.

f. Patients with severe congestive heart failure, post-myocardial infarction suspected to be related to papillary muscle dysfunction, ventricular septal defect or discrete aneurysm rather than global ventricular dysfunction.

The diversity of opinion concerning role of arteriography in the evaluation of patients with suspected or documented coronary disease, according to the same authors, is due to a combination of factors:

1. the continuing controversy over the role of coronary artery bypass surgery in the management of patients with ischaemic heart disease;

2. the invasive nature of the test and the attendant small but distinct morbidity and mortality; and

3. the fact that the quality of study and complication rate vary widely. In general, the performance record of laboratories doing less than 100 studies per year, for example, is not comparable with that of more active laboratories.

Angiographic visualization of deformity in the lumen of a vessel remains the best presumptive test of silent atherosclerosis. Coronary angiography now permits visualization and assessment of arteries as small as 0.5 mm in diameter.

Bypass Material

The predominant bypass material is the patient's own saphenous vein.

The saphenous vein of the lower leg usually has less valves and is similar in diameter to the coronary vessel compared to the vein of the upper thigh. Most surgeons remove the saphenous vein in total length selecting the best segments as bypass material. If the saphenous vein cannot be used, one of the arm veins can be utilized. Usually the arm veins are fragile, the wall being very thin.

An alternative to the patient's saphenous vein graft is his internal mammary artery. This is only used by about 10 to 20 per cent of the surgeons. This material is, however, more time-consuming to obtain and difficult to prepare. The internal mammary artery is able to provide enough flow for restoration of normal myocardial function and an excellent life time bypass graft. The diameter of the mammary artery increases in time. Reasons for the excellent longterm results of internal mammary artery bypass surgery, are that the vessel is an artery with a calibre very similar to that a coronary, thus less eddies and turbulence are expected at the site of anastomosis. There is thus a clear indication for the use of a mammary artery bypass graft in case the proper vein is not available.

During the dissection of the saphenous vein, any mechanical damage, like pinching by forceps or pulling on the vessel, has to be avoided.

Results of Bypass Surgery

The overall results of the bypass surgery have recently been analysed by different groups working in this field. Leclerc and his colleagues at the University of Alabama in Birmingham, U.S.A., analysed 6630 patients having coronary artery bypass grafting between August 1975 and December 1978 in 15 major medical centres in the United States and Canada, participating in the collaborative study in coronary artery surgery. They documented an overall operative mortality of 2.3 per cent. This mortality ranged from 0.3 per cent to 6.4 per cent among the 15 centres. Mortality for 5 elective surgery was 1.7 per cent, for urgent surgery was 3.5 per cent and for emergency surgery was 10.8 per cent. Old age, female sex, symptoms of heart failure, left main coronary artery stenosis, and impaired left ventricular function were the other factors associated with higher operative mortality rates.

Myocardial infarction at the time of operation (peri-operative myocardial infarction, POMI) was the most important fatal and non-fatal complication of the coronary bypass grafting procedure. With increasing surgical experience, there was a progressive decline in the incidence of this complication. For 1573 of 3057 patients having isolated coronary bypass grating at their hospital between January 1970 and December 1977, who had serial E.C.G. and enzymatic (SOT) data available for analysis, a progressive reduction in the annual incidence of infarction during the 8 year interval was observed. For 395 patients operated upon between January 1974 and December 1977, it was 2.4 per cent (28 patients), a highly significant difference. A major reduction was noted in 1974, coincident with modifications in anaesthetic management and myocardial protection, and despite an increase in the number of patients with multi-vessel disease undergoing operation, and in the number of grafts inserted per patient.

Congestive heart failure, presence of unstable angina, number of vessels diseased and the age of the patient, were the important predictors of peri-operative infarction.

Long-term Survival

The severity of preoperative left ventricular dysfunction, and, to a lesser extent, the severity of coronary artery disease are the most important determinants of long-term survival following bypass grafting. For patients with 50 per cent or greater narrowing of the left main coronary artery, survival following coronary artery bypass grafting exceeded that for non-operative therapy for virtually every identifiable subset of patients, and must be considered the treatment of choice. For patients with three vessel disease and essentially normal left ventricular function, several studies, demonstrated improved survival among surgically treated patients when compared to similar patients managed non-operatively.

Other results of the bypass surgery indicated that:

1. Surgical therapy is more effective in relieving severe angina pectoris than any currently available method of medical therapy. The number of patients free of angina decreased with

time, but the number of surgically treated patients who remained symptom-free, exceeded the number of medically treated patients for the first year.

2. Left ventricular performance improved.

3. Non-fatal ischaemic events are reduced.

4. Sudden death is reduced.

Sheldon and Loop at the Cleaveland Clinic Foundation, Ohio, U.S.A., analysed their 14-year experience in the bypass graft surgery in coronary artery disease. Their cases numbered 23853. The operative mortality, 8.6 per cent in 1967, declined to 1.4 per cent in 1973. The average number of grafts per patient increased from 1.5 in 1967-70 series to 2.6 per patient in 1980. In 1980, the overall operative mortality was 1.7 per cent and the cumulative mortality for 14 years was 2 per cent. Among 21,244 patients who were treated surgically till 1980 with bypass grafts exclusively, including emergency operations and reoperations, the cumulative mortality was 1.5 per cent (0.8 per cent for single grafts, 1.6 per cent for double grafts and 1.8 per cent for procedures involving 3 or more grafts). The rate of peri-operative infarction declined from 6.7 per cent in the series of patients operated upon in 1967-70 to 1.4 per cent in 1980. Operative mortality in patients with normal left ventricular function or only mild impairment of contractility fell from 2.7 per cent in the 1967-70 series to 1 per cent in a series of 1000 similar patients operated upon electively during the years 1971-1973. In patients with moderate left ventricular dysfunction, operative mortality fell from 3.3 per cent in the 1967-70 series to 1.5 per cent in the 1971-73 series.

Discussing their data, Sheldon and Loop said: "The accumulated experience of 14 years with bypass graft surgery, has led to better selection of patients, recognition of the importance of complete revascularization, improved operative and peri-operative management with myocardial preservation technics, mechanical circulatory assistance in selected cases, diminution of blood requirement, and more effective pharmacologic support. As a result, operative mortality is lower and medium and long-term survival is better, especially of patients with more extensive disease."

At the Montreal Heart Institute, Quebec, Canada, a study was made of the fate of bypass graft. Campeau and his colleagues concluded that "the most important determinants of early graft patency appear to be the quality of the distal run off and surgical techniques. We have shown that patency at one year may be as high as 89.7 per cent in graft to arteries with good distal runoff and as low as 44 per cent when the distal coronary segment is inadequate. Optimal surgical techniques involving the excision and preparation of the saphenous vein, anastomoses and the designs for the bypasses also appear to determine graft patency. Early graft patency attrition is also related to contraction of anastomoses which may be due to inadequate surgical techniques or to an excessively small grafted artery. The patency did not appear to be influenced by the degree of the preoperative obstruction on the coronary artery segment proximal to the graft anastomosis, the quality of wall motion in the area of the grafted artery, the quality of the vein, nor to serum lipid abnormalities."

Bypass Closure: Causes

Studies of aorto-coronary vein grafts obtained from patients surviving the operation for periods up to 5 years have indicated that thrombosis, intimal proliferative changes and the development of atherosclerosis are the main processes affecting the integrity of the graft. In addition, factors such as technical considerations in performing the proximal and distal anastomosis, placing grafts too small, diseased coronary arteries with limited distal vascular beds, degree of proximal stenosis, and elevated blood lipids, may contribute to saphenous vein occlusion. During the first two months following surgery, thrombosis accounts for most occlusions, whereas by one year, obstruction results principally from slowly progressive intimal fibrous reaction. Ulcreated plaques, cholesterol clefts and focal haemorrhage, the hall-mark of overt atherosclerosis were present in nearly one-third to one-half of the graft recovered 3 years or more after operation. Thus the spectrum of graft abnormalities that determine its patency is rather wide and changes with time after surgery. It is unlikely that one factor determines the course of changes in the vascular graft and in the adjacent coronary artery

Some authors have presented evidence that a "hypercoagulable state" is involved in thrombotic graft occlusion. Anti-coagulant therapy has been shown to prevent and limit thrombosis of peripheral veins. It would, therefore, offer a potential way to affect the occurrence of thrombosis in saphenous vein grafts. In addition, Steele and his colleagues have shown that a relationship between shortened platelet survival and graft occlusion exists and these authors have suggested that platelet function inhibiting drugs might be useful in preventing graft closure.

Bypass Surgery: Latest Opinion

According to Braunwald and Cohn (1983), certain areas of agreement about the bypass surgery can be identified:

1. The operation is relatively safe, with reported mortality rates as low as 1 per cent in elective operations carried out by experienced surgical teams in patients with normal or near normal left ventricular function.

2. Operative and post-operative mortality increases with left ventricular dysfunction and with surgical inexperience.

3. The graft procedure is surgically feasible, with patency rates of 70 to 80 per cent reported at 2 to 3 years. Ultimate patency of the graft correlates with graft flow at the time of operation. The frequency of occlusion of grafts with flow rates exceeding 50 ml/min is very low.

4. Grafts that become occluded usually do so within 1 year.

5. When a bypass operation is performed on a partially occluded vessel, the probability of the partial obstruction in the native circulation progressing to completion is markedly increased.

6. Angina is unequivocally relieved in 85 per cent of patients, although drug therapy may still be necessary in many. In most instances, this relief can be attributed to increased blood flow to the ischaemic myocardium, but this is not an adequate explanation in all patients. For example, relief of symptoms in the presence of occluded grafts could be due to infarction of the ischaemic or angina-producing segment of the myocardium. The well-known placebo effect of operation is another possible mechanism for symptomatic improvement, but relief due to this mechanism would not be expected to be long-lasting. The fact that symptomatic relief

95

is attributable to increased flow is also supported by the occasional fortuitous arteriographic demonstration that pain abruptly recurs when a graft becomes occluded, suggesting that the placebo effect is not entirely responsible for the relief of pain.

7. The inability to demonstrate ventriculographic or hemodynamic improvement of global ventricular function after bypass operation in some patients is not surprising when it is recognized that improvement could not be expected in those patients who have normal ventricular function prior to operation, or in patients with ventricular function impaired by previous infarction and scar or aneurysm formation.

8. Peri-operative and intra-operative myocardial infarction occurs in 8 to 15 per cent of patients. In most instances these infarcts are small.

9. The mortality rate of patients with unoperated left main coronary artery lesions is exceedingly high, and the results of some studies suggest that this rate can be reduced by operative intervention.

10. The mortality of patients with unoperated single vessel disease limited either to the circumflex or right coronary arteries is low and does not differ greatly from that of age-matched controls without any disease.

The objective of surgical treatment include the relief of symptoms and improvement of exercise tolerance, improvement of ventricular function, prevention of myocardial infarction, and improvement of life expectancy. The impressive ability of the procedure to relieve pain in most patients is a remarkable feature.

An important factor in the bypass operation relates to the technical sklls of the surgical and diagnostic teams, and the quality of care in post-operative period. As a general rule, the poorest results are reported from institutions performing the least number of operations, and the advisability of having operation carried out by an experienced surgical team cannot be over emphasized.

Asymptomatic Coronary Atherosclerosis

According to Selwyn and Braunwald (1986), the widespread use of exercise stress test during routine annual examination, has shown evidence of silent myocardial ischaemia, i.e. exercise induced electrocardiographic changes not accompanied by angina. Coronary angiography in such persons frequently reveal obstructive coronary artery disease. Post-mortem studies in patients with obstructive coronary artery disease who had no history of myocardial ischaemia frequently showed macroscopic scars of myocardial infarction in regions supplied by diseased coronary arteries.

In addition, population studies have shown that approximately 25 per cent of patients with acute myocaridal infarctions may not reach medical attention, and that these carry the same adverse prognosis as those in whom the symptoms of ischaemia develop.

Patients who are asymptomatic after an infarct are nonetheless at greater risk for a second coronary event than the general population. Although medical therapy (elimination of smoking, antihypertensive medication, diet, etc.) aimed at preventing progression of surgery improves mortality in coronary patients have led some to advocate routine coronary arteriography to establish a diagnosis and subsequent bypass surgery if anatomically feasible despite the asymptomatic state.

Bypass Operation in Acute Evolving Myocardial Infarction (AEMI)

Infarction is not an instantaneous occurrence. It involves the passage of time. It is now realized that patient in the acute evolving myocardial infarction syndrome have reversibly damaged myocardium which can be salvaged by prompt restoration of blood flow.

Ralphberg, Selinger and Leonard at Sacred Heart Medical Centre in Deaconess Hospital, Spokane, U.S.A. reported one such study. From March 1971 through April 1980, 260 patients underwent immediate coronary bypass for AEMI. All the patients fulfilled the criteria for AEMI as follow:

1. Chest pain typical of infarction.

2. Q wave greater than 0.04 seconds in duration and ST injury pattern in E.C.G.

3. Major lesions greater than 90 per cent on coronary artery cineangiography.

4. Ventriculographic abnormality.

5. Elevation of SGOT and creatinine kinase.

Mortality for conventional management of AEMI patients was 11.5 per cent for the first 30 days. This group of 260 patients receiving coronary bypass had a 2.3 per cent in hospital mortality. The first year mortality plus one year mortality with conventional management exceeded 30 per cent, while the sum of 3.5 per cent for surgical management yielded roughly a nine fold difference in the two methods.

Cardiac Rehabilitation after Bypass Surgery

Cardiac rehabilitation after bypass surgery includes the reconditioning of the patient with the improvement of physical exercise performance and the counselling of the patient.

Most patients stay after the bypass operation for a total of 8 weeks for cardiac rehabilitation and participate in a graded exercise programme that is adjusted to the individual's age and activity status before surgery.

The exercise programme begins with the usual passive exercise on the first operative day. At seven days, the patient walks in the hallways and climbs one flight of stairs with a physiotherapist monitoring the heart rate. At two weeks, an endurance exercise training at a low work load is started on a bicycle ergometer with central monitoring of the heart rate. The average work load after two weeks would be 25 watts for 2 minutes, followed by a break of one minute, again followed by 2 minutes exercise. After a second break of one minute, the work load is increased to 50 watts and continued for another 2 minutes. This kind of exercise is done five times a week. At four weeks after the surgery, an exercise test at the 50 watt level in the supine position is performed. During the next four weeks, the endurance training is gradually increased and includes walking in water with E.C.G. monitoring; after 7 to 8 weeks, a symptom-limited exercise test in the supine position with measurement of pulmonary capillary wedge pressure and estimation of cardiac output is performed. The effect of training is reflected in the decrease of the resting morning heart rate.

The marked decrease of the resting heart rate and the decrease of the heart rate at the given work load between 4 and 8 weeks after surgery, reflects improved conditioning during the post-operative period.

Coronary Bypas Surgery in India

Coronary bypass surgery (CBS) is at present performed in different centres in India. (See Useful addresses)

The operations are done after proper assessment of the cases, the most important part of which is the coronary angiography. The CBS operation is performed in cases of angina pectoris and those who have had a previous heart attack. Improvement is observed after the operation in 70 to 80 per cent of the cases. These results are comparable with those obtained in the Western countries.

Life expectancy is increased after CBS surgery particularly in those cases having left (main) coronary artery disease. Mortality at or around the time of operation is 3 to 4 per cent. This figure is higher than that obtained outside India where it is between 1 to 2 per cent.

Those centres where more CBS operations are done, have gradually over the years improved their results because of the following reasons:

1. Longer experience of the operating surgeons.
2. Longer experience of the paramedical staff like nurses, etc.
3. Better team-work.
4. Better post-operative care.
5. Adequate and up-to-date equipment.

The cost to the patient in India for the CBS operation differs from centre to centre from Rs 20,000 to Rs 50,000. Abroad this comes to Rs 2 to 3 hundred thousands (Rs 2 to 3 lakhs). The stay in the hospital in uncomplicated cases in India varies from 10 days to 2 weeks.

A regular follow-up of the operated cases is an important feature. On this score, the patients that are operated upon in India in centres near their homes, are at an advantage. This is because of the convenience of shorter distance and less expenditure involved. It is certain that very soon, even the rich and well-connected patients, would not feel the need to travel abroad for this operation.

Transluminal Coronary Angioplasty

Another type of surgical procedure done in patients having coronary artery narrowing and its consequential effects, is transluminal coronary angioplasty.

In 1964, Dotter and Judkins in Portland, Oregon, U.S.A., introduced a new therapeutic catheter technique designed to improve flow in peripheral arteries with obstructive arteriosclerosis. This method was termed "transluminal angioplasty". Following their pioneering work, Gruentzig in Zurich developed a double-lumen catheter which employed at its distal end a destensible balloon with a fixed outer diameter when inflated. Since 1974, when used in the leg arteries, the Gruentzing angioplasty system achieved an initial patency of 86 per cent and a three year cumulative patency of 73 per cent.

In 1976, Gruentzig miniaturized his peripheral angioplasty catheter system to perform coronary angioplasty, first in experimental dogs and subsequently in human cadavers. In 1977, in San Francisco and Zurich, Gruentzig and Myler first performed angioplasty to assess its applicability in living human atherosclerosis. Subsequently Gruentzig first performed percutaneous transluminal coronary angioplasty (PTCA) in the cardiac catheterization laboratory at the University Hospital, Zurich, and two months later PTCA was performed in Frankfurt with Dr. Kaltenbach.

In March 1978, PTCA was introduced to the United States by Myler and Stertzer. Recently PTCA has been reported in 1000 patients in 58 centres throughout the world and submitted to the National Heart, Lung, Blood Institute, registry for PTCA, at the National Institute of Health.

Materials: To perform PTCA, at present the equipment consists of two catheters and a calibrated pressure pump. The larger catheter, termed the guiding catheter (GC) is a bonded composite of three layers. The dilatation catheter (DC) consists of two lumina, a central one for pressure measurements and supraselective control injection, and an eccentric lumen for balloon inflation/deflation. The balloon is made of polyvinychloride and is located at the distal tip of the D.C. It is 2.0 cm long and either 3.0 or 3.7 mm in outer diameter when inflated (for use in standard coronary arteries or saphenous vein grafts respectively for example). The pressure pump is calibrated.

Methods: After routine coronary arteriography to evaluate the present anatomic and pathologic status of patients (previously selected by arteriography and clinical status for PTCA), the GC is inserted and advanced over a guide wire into the ascending aorta and then into the appropriate coronary artery opening. The D.C. is then passed through GC to emerge in the coronary artery.

The D.C. is then advanced with continuous pressure monitoring and intermittent contrast injection into the coronary artery selected for angioplasty. Careful positioning of the D.C. is obviously necessary to insure intraluminal location and placement of the balloon at the site of stenosis. When properly positioned, the balloon is inflated 2-4 times at 4-6 atmospheres for approximately 15 seconds for each inflation/deflation cycle. With successful angioplasty, a rise in the pressure is recorded and improved run off contrast in the vessel distally visualized.

Subsequently the D.C. is withdrawn, recording the final pullback pressure gradient, and then is removed through the GC. Post-angioplasty coronary arteriography is then obtained in precisely the same planes and obliquities as recorded in the control study.

Medical therapy for PTCA includes nitrates by various routes (including intracoronary) and calcium antagonists to diminish the tendency to coronary spasm, and platelet inhibitors to decrease platelet response, both predictable consequences of angioplasty.

After successful coronary angioplasty, the patient is returned to a monitored unit for 24-hour observation. If no untoward events are noticed, the patient is discharged the following day.

Results: From 58 centres in the United States and Europe, 1000 patients were evaluated. Of these, 79 per cent were male, 21 per cent female with an age range of 23-76 years, (means 51 years).

The average duration of angina in this series was 15 months, with a range of less than one month to more than ten years. In these 1000 patients, 78 per cent had single-vessel coronary artery disease, 16 per cent double vessel disease, 4 per cent triple-vessel disease and 2 per cent left main coronary artery disease.

In 1053 arteries attempted in these 1000 patients, 65 per cent involved the left anterior descending coronary artery, 25 per cent the right coronary artery, the 5 per cent left circumflex and 2 per cent left (main) and 3 per cent were attempted in saphenous vein grafts. In these 1053 coronary arteries, successful angioplasty (defined as luminal diameter improvement of greater than 20 per cent) was achieved in 59 per cent. Twelve per cent of the lesions were "too hard" to dilate and in another 29 per cent, the D.C. could not cross the lumen, either because the lesion was too stenotic to allow passage or because of peculiarities in the coronary anatomy.

Analyzed by vessel, successful angioplasty was performed in 71 per cent of 21 left main coronary lesions, 35 per cent of 55 left circumflex lesions, 56 per cent of 261 right coronary lesions and 61 per cent of 33 saphenous vein grafts. It was noted that experience brought better results so that recent operations showed better results than earlier ones.

In these 1000 cases, there were 13 (1.3 per cent) hospital deaths. All of these patients underwent emergency coronary artery bypass grafting (CABG) after complicated PTCA. Emergency CABG was necessary in 64 (6 per cent) of patients. Myocardial infarction was noted in 48 (6 per cent) and ventricular fibrillation occurred in 14 (5 per cent) of patients. Further analysis of the mortality rate revealed 6 deaths in 769 patients with single-vessle disease (0.7 per cent) and 7 deaths in 196 patients multi-vessel disease (3.6 per cent). In patients without prior CABG, there were 5 deaths in 728 (0.8 per cent), and 2 deaths in 163 patients (1.2 per cent), respectively. It is noteworthy that in more experienced centres for PTCA, there was a significant fall in the complication rate commensurate with the rise in success rate.

Initial one-year PTCA follow-up in successfully treated patients revealed improvement in 83 per cent, no change in 6 per cent and worsening in 1 per cent. Repeat PTCA was performed in 4 per cent, CABG in 5 per cent and repeat PTCA and CABG in 1 per cent.

Discussing the subject, Myler, Gruentzing and others stated the situation regarding the PTCA as follows:

Presently we would recommend PTCA in patients with subjective and objective evidence of myocardial ischaemia who have failed optimal medical management and are candidates for CABG. Of course, they must have lesions which are suitable for angioplasty—discrete, subtotal and relatively concentric lesions which are not calcified and do not involve major branch bifurcations. The anatomic limitations of coronary angioplasty are generally those of lesion accessibility. Tortuous vessels, sharp angulations, multiple branches proximal to the lesions and cul-de-sac lesions all may inhibit successful angioplasty. It appears that the shorter the anginal history, especially in lesions involving the left anterior descending coronary artery, the greater the expectation of a successful angioplasty.

Although single-vessel coronary artery disease is preferred for PTCA, because successful angioplasty should normalize subjective and objective parameters of myocardial ischaemia, angioplasty has been performed in carefully selected patients with multivessel coronary artery disease. These are either post-CABG patients in whom one vessel will be attempted, or are patients in whom other diseased vessels are unsuitable for CABG. Totally occluded vessels are generally not attempted unless the occlusion is very recent, and there is no evidence of acute infarction. Left 'main' coronary artery lesions have been attempted. A significant percentage of the overall mortality has been noted in this group. At present we would recommend PTCA in patients with left 'main' coronary artery disease, who have isolated lesions, are post-CABG or in emergency conditions, e.g. cardiogenic shock. Saphenous vein graft steonsis are recommended in patients operated upon within one year prior to PTCA. The cause of this type of stenosis is often technical, leading to an inflammatory stenosis. Sustained patency in the small series of saphenous vein graft stenosis submitted to angioplasty has been lower than in native coronary vessels, which have undergone PTCA.

It would appear that PTCA is an effective treatment for selected patients with coronary arteriosclerosis who would otherwise be candidates for CABG because of subjective and objective evidence of myocardial ischaemia and relative refractoriness of medical therapy. The relatively low incidence of abrupt reclosure requiring CABG (5 per cent), the low mortality rate (1 per cent), and the noted restenosis rate of 12-16 per cent even with this preliminary experience with coronary angioplasty, would also indicate that this procedure is relatively safe.

Risks: More than one vessel can be dilated in sequence with a modest increase in risk. In female sex, the presence of left ventricular damage, a stenosis of an artery which perfuses a large segment of myocardium without collaterals, long irregular stenosis, and calcified plaques, all increase the likelihood of complications.

The major complications are usually due to dissection or thrombosis with vessel occlusion, uncontrolled ischaemia, and ventricular failure. In the most experienced hands, the overall mortality rate is less than 1 per cent, the need for emergency coronary surgery 3 to 5 per cent, and myocardial infarction in approximately 3 per cent of patients.

Reopening of the blocked or narrowed coronaries

An obstructing or nearly obstructing thrombus overlying or adjacent to an atherosclerotic plaque in a coronary artery, appears to be the cause of most myocardial infarcts. Therefore, reperfusion of the ischaemic zone by the prompt dissolution of the thrombus with a thrombolytic agent is a logical approach to the reduction of infarct size. There is considerable evidence that if reperfusion is to be effective in salvaging jeopardized myocardium, it must be carried out immediately after the onset of the clinical event; certainly within 4 hours and preferably within 2 hours.

According to Selwyn and Braunwald (1986), streptokinase (SK) given via a coronary catheter in the treatment of acute myocardial infarction, proved effective in lysing, the offending thrombus in about 75 per cent of cases. But whether this procedure reduces mortality or morbidity is not yet certain. It needs to be studied.

Another thrombus - dissolving agent called tissue plasminogen activator (tpa) has also been used intravenously. It caused lysis in approximately two-thirds of recent coronary thrombi. It has the theoretical advantage of causing fibrinolytic activity predominently at the site of a fresh thrombus, and thus may be safer than streptokinase by virtue of causing a less intensive systemic lytic state.

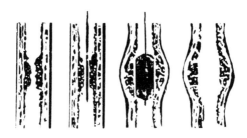

Fig. 14   Reopening of the Blocked Coronary

Whether thrombolytic therapy will be effective in routinely salvaging myocardium, whether mechanical revascularization by means of coronary angioplasty or coronary bypass surgery will be required following successful thrombolysis in the majority of patients and whether the mortality and morbidity of acute myocardial infarction can actually be reduced by this intervention, is still to be seen and analysed.

9

Prevention of Heart Attack

H eart attacks can be prevented by preventing the development of atherosclerosis in the coronary arteries. Let us recapitulate how this atherosclerosis occurs. Besides other factors, the occurrence of atherosclerosis depends on the level of cholesterol in the blood. The level of cholesterol depends upon the intake of cholesterol and fats in the diet.

Diet Control

Diet control is therefore of prime importance. Of the dietary fats, the unsaturated ones (derived from vegetable sources), not only do not increase the level of cholesterol, but also lessen it.

Taking into view the above findings, the American Heart Association, 1961, recommended three methods of reducing cholesterol in the blood:

1. Reduce the total amount of food taken.
2. Reduce the percentage of calories derived from fat.
3. Change the type of fats taken from the saturated animal type to the unsaturated vegetable type.

These then are the diet methods by observing which we can reduce the incidence of atherosclerosis of the coronary arteries and of heart attacks.

In order to follow these methods, let us first have a look at some of the common articles in our diet and see the quantity and quality of fats contained in them and how they affect blood cholesterol level and the coronary arteries.

Milk: It contains fats most of which come under the saturated category. The lesser the fat content of milk, the better it is for the coronaries. Skimmed milk is the best in this regard.

So is the case with milk products. *Ghee* (clarified butter) or butter (made from milk)—most of it being saturated fat—is not good for the coronaries, even though it may be good for the rest of the body. Hence, as little of it should be taken as possible.

Butter-milk (*mattha*) or whey (*lassi*) which is made from curd (from which fat has been churned out) is very good for the coronaries.

Meat, poultry and fish: Parts of meat devoid of fat may be taken in moderation. Ordinary mutton prepared in *desi ghee* (clarified butter) taken many times a week is detrimental to the coronary arteries because the fats in it are of the saturated variety. As a precaution, one should remove the crust of fat on the cold meat curry, and then warm it and take it.

Chicken contains less of saturated fat; it also contains some unsaturated fats—more than what mutton or beef contains.

There is no restriction on taking fish. Fish contains less of fat and whatever fat it contains, is highly unsaturated. Rather than raising it, fish lessens blood cholesterol.

Organ meat such as liver, kidneys, brain contains large amount of cholesterol. Hence, they may be avoided.

Eggs: Yellow of the eggs contains a lot of cholesterol, hence eggs must be taken in moderation, not more than two or three a week for a normal healthy person. But those who have the coronary heart disease, or have high blood cholesterol level, it is better that they avoid taking eggs.

The cholesterol content (mg per 100 gms) of the following articles of diet is: brain 2,000; egg yolk 1,500; liver 600; pork 600; kidneys 400; butter 300; lobster 300; shrimp 150; crab 150; cheese 150; beef 110; fish (most) 50; vegetables 0.

Hydrogenated fats and oils: Hydrogenated fat or what goes by the name of vegetable *ghee,* contains a high percentage of saturated

107

solid fat converted from unsaturated liquid oils. These are unhealthy for the coronary arteries.

On the other hand, vegetable oils such as ground-nut oil, mustard, sesame (*til*) oil, safflower oil and sunflower oil, contain a lot of unsaturated fat, and are good for the coronaries.

There is an exception among the oils: coconut oil contains too much of saturated fat and hence is not good for coronaries.

Vegetable oils, in common use in India, have the following percentage of saturated and unsaturated fats:

Oil	Sat. fat %	Unsat. fat %
Safflower	8	55
Sesame	14	44
Cotton seed	25	50
Ground-nut	20	26
Coconut	86	0
Hydrogenated fat	High	0

Vegetarian Diet: People who take a vegetarian diet have lower serum cholesterol level than those who are non-vegetarians. The substitution of vegetable oil for animal fats (without change in fat content or total calories), reduces serum cholesterol level.

The benefit of vegetable diet is related to the presence of the plant sterol, sitosterol, which lowers blood cholesterol. It is found to decrease the incidence of atherosclerosis in cholesterol-fed rabbits and chicks. Sitosterol probably acts by interfering with the absorption of dietary cholesterol and cholesterol excreted by the liver into the intestines.

Vegetables contain no cholesterol. Different types of cereals also contain no cholesterol and they contain some unsaturated fats as well. Onion and garlic can be used; some people have found them to be useful for the coronaries. Different types of nuts, such as walnuts, almonds, ground-nuts, contain a fair amount of unsaturated fats and are good for the coronaries.

Practical Hints on Diet: Omit or curtail drastically the intake of egg yolk, fatty meat, butter, whole milk, cream, ice-cream, creamed foods, gravies, fatty soups, chocolates and cakes.

Substitute vegetable oil for *ghee* or hydrogenated *ghee*, skimmed milk for whole milk, fish and poultry for mutton and pork.

• Take more of seasonal fruits and cooked or raw vegetables.

• Take lesser amount of total food in a day.

• Such a diet—containing low calories, and less fat (that too of unsaturated type)—should be taken by all those who have:

1. High blood cholesterol level
2. Hypertension
3. Diabetes
4. Overweight
5. Family history of heart attacks
6. All those who wish to live a long healthy life without the overhanging danger of heart attacks.

Since it takes long decades over which the coronaries get narrowed, these precautions in diet should be observed not only by adults or middle-aged people but children also. Habits formed in childhood are naturally carried on in adult life.

Cholesterol-reducing Drugs: Nicotinic acid can lower the level of blood cholesterol but not without producing side-effects such as loss of hair, scaly skin, flushing. A variant of nicotinic acid does not cause flushing, but causes instead stomach upset and ulcers.

Reduce High Blood Pressure

Many people think they can tell high blood pressure is present by headaches or other symptoms. The fact is that the only way to know if the blood pressure is raised is by having it measured by blood-pressure measuring apparatus—sphygmomanometer. Blood pressure, which is higher than normal, causes excessive stretching of the blood vessel wall and hastens its wear and tear. It accelerates the process of atherosclerosis. Other factors aside, people with high blood pressure are reported to have five times more heart attacks than those who have normal blood pressure.

Salt Intake and Blood Pressure: In large majority of patients who have high blood pressure, it is not yet possible to find out the cause of the condition; the condition is thus labelled as Essential

Hypertension, though there is nothing essential about it. In these patients, however, some interesting observations have been made about their habit of eating salt (common table salt: sodium chloride).

In early 1950s, a large number of men were checked about the quantity of salt that they took in their diet and their blood pressure. These people were divided into three groups: in the first group were those who never salted their food (yet it contained 2 to 3 gms of salt as a constituent of daily diet); second, who took 4 to 10 gms. of salt a day; and third, who took 12 to 18 gms of salt.

It was found that in the high-salt group, 10 per cent people had hypertension; in the moderate salt group, 7 per cent had hypertension, and in the low salt group, there was no case of hypertension.

This finding was subsequently confirmed by animal experiments. Two groups of rats were put on high and low salt. The high salt group developed hypertension; when out of this group, some of the rats were put on even higher salt diet, their blood pressure increased further.

It has been found that hypertensive patients, on the whole, feel satisfied about the adequateness of salt in their diet only when there is a higher than ordinary content of it in it.

The above studies indicate that high salt content in the diet increases blood pressure. The converse is also true in many cases of hypertension: lowering salt content of their diet lowers their blood pressure.

Lowering salt content in the diet or even omitting it altogether has no adverse effect upon health. Actually, there is enough natural salt in the vegetables and other foods including milk. In the past, salt was not available to people living in many areas of the world. In our country, many sadhus and ascetics are known to abstain from taking salt for years together. They are none the worse for it; in fact, they say they enjoy better health because of lack of salt.

As a result of the above observations, many pharmaceutical firms have come up with drugs that increase the passage of salt in the urine, thereby depleting the body of the salt which the patient has taken. Unfortunately, however, with the salt (sodium chloride) other essential salts are also drained out in the process, so that the patient feels weak and has other side-effects.

Thus, we see that in order to lower blood pressure, it is better to use less salt in the diet and not to depend upon drugs to do this job.

Foods particularly high in salt are: pickles, *chutnies,* canned or bottled soups and vegetables, sausages, hot dogs, ham, bacon, salted nuts, popcorn, potato chips.

Alkalizers taken for stomach upset, e.g. Eno's fruit salt, and even chewing tobacco have excess salt.

In order to limit the salt intake:

1. Don't put salt in any article of food at the table;
2. Take the help of different spices to remove the bland taste in unsalted diet.

Other Blood Pressure Reducing Measures: If hypertension is mild but persistent, the patient is advised to reduce his weight if he is overweight. Giving a mild sedative or a tranquilliser may bring it down to normal in a few weeks.

In case the blood pressure is high, besides the above precautions, one may need to take a drug or a combination of drugs.

The patient has to realise that once drug treatment is embarked upon, it will need to be continued for life at least in the present state of our knowledge. The establishment of a good relationship between the doctor and the patient is very important. The previously asymptomatic patient who develops side-effects of treatment needs particular help: appropriate adjustment of the dose, or change of drug may restore his confidence. The treatment has to be reviewed regularly; whether the supervision should be by a general practitioner or by hospital doctors with a special interest in hypertension, depends on many factors and let be decided by the patient.

Approach to Drug Therapy: The aim of drug therapy is to use the drugs alone or in combination, to return arterial pressure to normal levels with minimal side-effects. When used in combination, drugs should be chosen for their different sites of action. Those who have higher blood pressure (average diastolic pressure 130 mm Hg or more) will require more intensive therapy with several drugs simultaneously.

For those patients requiring multiple drugs, once the appropriate combination has been found, the use of a single pill with the appropriate combination of drugs may simplify the regimen and thereby increase compliance. Every effort should be made to reduce the number of times each day the patient must interrupt his or her schedule for the medication.

Probably fewer than one-third of the diagnosed hypertensive patients get treated effectively. Only a small number of these failures is related to drug unresponsiveness. The majority is related to:

1. failure to institute effective treatment of the asymptomatic hypertensive subject, and

2. failure of the asymptomatic hypertensive subject to adhere to therapy.

In order to improve this deficiency, patients must be educated to continue treatment once an effective regimen has been identified. Side-effects and inconveniences of treatment must be minimised or counteracted in order to obtain the patients' continued cooperation.

Combined with moderate salt restriction, diuretic pills are effective in lowering blood pressure, initially by reducing blood volume, and over a longer period by reducing peripheral arteriolar resistance, probably in part by removing salt from the arterial wall. They are particularly useful for minor degrees of hypertension. Many have the disadvantage of causing excessive potassium loss. A cheap long-acting thiazide diuretic together with potassium supplement is helpful. Rapidly acting diuretics such as frusemide are less useful, unless there is accompanying heart or kidney failure. Diuretics are also a useful adjunct to other forms of treatment.

Of the sympatholytic drugs, the beta-adrenergic receptor blocking drugs are now the most widely used. Propranolol is effective and its reliability and relative freedom from side-effects appears to be established. The dose has to be adjusted to the individual's need. The combination of propranolol and a diuretic usually with a potassium supplement achieves the therapeutic goal without significant side-effects in a high proportion of patients with essential hypertension.

If this proves not to be the case, other sympatholytic agents may be effective. Clonidine, starting with 0.1 mg three times a day and rising to 1 mg in total per day, has a predominantly central action. Methyldopa, starting with 250 mg three times a day and rising to 3 gm total per day, has both a central and peripheral action.

Control of Diabetes

Heart attacks are common in diabetic patients, and they have them at a comparatively younger age. Women who have diabetes suffer heart attack more often than normals.

Diabetes (or diabetes mellitus, as its full name is) is characterised by high level of sugar (glucose) in the blood so that some of this sugar filters out of the kidneys in the urine.

High level of glucose in the blood is due to the fact that the food that we take and which consists of proteins, fats and carbohydrates, is converted after digestion and absorption into glucose and enters the blood. This glucose in the blood is used up for supplying energy to the body for its various activities, and the spare amount of glucose is converted into glycogen so that it can be stored up in the muscles and the liver for any future use.

Glucose is converted into glycogen with the help of insulin, a secretion of the pancreas which is situated a little below the stomach, on the left side in the upper abdomen.

If for certain reasons, the secretion of insulin is less than is needed by the body, then much of glucose remains as such in the blood and after filtering through the kidneys, flows out with the urine.

A diabetic patient feels easily fatigued because the food that he takes and which is converted in the body into glucose, flows out of the urine and is wasted. Less of glycogen is stored in the body so that at the time of physical exertion, extra glucose is not available and the patient feels fatigued easily.

As a result of disturbance in the glucose metabolism, more fats are broken down in the body to provide energy to it and more of them flow in the bloodstream. Cholesterol level in the blood is raised and there are atherosclerotic changes in the coronary arteries and blood vessels of the brain and the kidneys.

Diabetes is a very common disease. It is said that almost one per cent of the population in India suffers from it. Those who are obese and those who eat more and take a more nutritious diet, suffer from it more. That is why its incidence is higher in people living in countries where the standard of living (and eating) is much higher.

Diabetes may be present in the young as well as the old; its prevalence is the highest after the middle age, almost equally in both the sexes.

Diabetic people are more prone to heart attacks. They are also the people who are generally overweight and have hypertension which makes them susceptible to heart attacks.

Even people who are in pre-diabetic stage, i.e. those who may not be passing sugar in the urine and yet have more than normal glucose in their blood, or those who on testing (glucose tolerance test) are found not to turn glucose into glycogen adequately so that their blood sugar rises higher than it does in the normal people, are also more susceptible to heart attacks. Such people are generally the relations of diabetic people.

Diabetes can be controlled either by proper diet alone, or by proper diet plus drugs. If a person is overweight, he must shed extra kilograms that he has. This by itself may bring diabetes under control.

If this does not happen, the patient needs to consult a competent doctor who, after doing all the necessary tests, can put him on proper drugs and other management measures.

Diabetes must be kept under proper control to minimise damage to the coronary arteries and to the heart.

Reduce Extra Weight

Life insurance statistics from the U.S.A. show that mortality from heart attack in overweight people is 40 per cent higher than among normal-weight people.

A person is considered overweight when his weight exceeds 10 per cent of what it ideally should be, taking into consideration the height and built of the person.

Weight of the body is normally maintained by two factors:

1. the amount of food we take, and

2. the amount of energy we spend in our day-to-day living.

The food that we take is converted in the body into calories. (A calorie is the measure of the amount of heat or energy which the body derives from a given amount of food). Normally, the calories produced from the food we eat, are spent in our day-to-day living.

If, however, we take more food calories than we spend—or even though we do not eat in excess, and yet spend less calories in our day-to-day activities—the calories not spent remain stored inside the body in the form of fat. If the process goes on, more and more fat is accumulated and extra weight is put on. This makes clear an apparently paradoxical situation in which a person says that he eats very little food and yet he is putting on weight. Or, may be he is eating more than he is aware of! If you ask him to write down each and every bit of edible thing that he takes, not only you, but he himself will be astonished at the things which he eats but which don't register in his mind.

In a majority of the cases it is falsely believed that obesity is inherited in the family. Obesity in more than one member in a family is due to the common habit of overeating that prevails in the family.

Neither it is due to hormonal imbalance or defect in the thyroid. Those who increase in weight even on low-diet, do so because they have the habit of spending less energy, i.e. they are physically less active.

All obese people wish to reduce weight because of various reasons: obese persons do not look pretty or handsome; they suffer more from diabetes, high blood pressure, heart attacks, aches and pains in joints, are more prone to accidents, and are liable to die earlier than many other people of their age group. But in spite of the wish being there, they do not reduce weight because either they do not know how to do it or they do not have the will to do so.

It is not that people who are overweight do not know or do not care about the frightening prospects ahead. Most of them would tell you over a tea-party or a dinner that they are on a 'reducing diet.' However, while ladies may take half a teaspoonful of sugar in their tea, they do not hesitate to gulp down one or more pastries, and an overweight gentleman prefers to take tea without sugar but does not mind relishing a full *tandoori murga*. No wonder when you meet such people year after year, they have increased in weight, though they have been on a 'diet'.

There are more fads and fancies about how to reduce weight than perhaps about all other things put together. There are fads about taking a single article of food such as curd, skimmed milk, tomato juice, spinach, etc. twice or thrice a day for a month or so. There are fads against certain foods such as potatoes and sugar because of their alleged fattening effect. Then there are fads about taking only uncooked articles of foods.

If an overweight person wants to reduce his weight, he must either eat less, or he must spend more calories in daily activities such as regular physical exercise. Ideally, he should do both the things together: eat less and spend more calories in extra physical activity.

The first essential of the diet for reducing weight should be that it is tasty enough to be adopted as a regular diet, not for a day, a month, or a year, but for all time to come. It should be so varied that the person eating it feels satisfied and does not tire out of it. It should be a balanced diet containing proteins, fats, carbohydrates, vitamins, minerals and water, in the right proportion to each other. Such a diet should include ordinary food stuffs, the kind taken by the family. It should consist of milk, fruits, vegetables, cereals and some quantity of fat. It should not contain the so called party dishes, i.e. those that are fried.

To lose half a kg. of body weight, an average adult must lose 3,500 calories spread over a week. This can be achieved by daily consuming food of 500 calories less. A better method would be to cut down the intake of 250-300 calories, and by spending 150 to 250 calories more in physical exercise, such as, brisk walking, running, cycling, swimming, gardening or playing some strenuous game.

Some practical suggestions with regard to eating are as follows:

Eat slowly. In this way the appetite centre in the brain gets satisfied before you have taken more food than you really need.

Masticate your food thoroughly. This helps in making smaller meals more satisfying.

Omit a second helping. Some people find it difficult to refuse second helpings when they are dining out. This is due more to lack of will power and resolution than to politeness.

Have a weighing machine in your house and take your weight daily before breakfast. See how much you wanted to reduce and how much you have. On the basis of that reading, chalk out your programme of eating for the day, i.e. whether you should eat less of a meal. Use of a weighing machine for an obese patient is as important as is that of a thermometer for a patient having high fever.

Do not skip meals. You will soon feel more hungry and then may eat even more.

Do not aim to reduce more than 1/2 kg. per week. Rapid weight-reduction in a coronary patient may actually precipitate an heart attack. During very rapid weight reduction, utilisation of the patient's own fat is tantamount to a high fat diet.

Control community eating. If you have to dine out on a particular day, eat less during the day.

You can dull your appetite before meals by taking initially a glass of water or a good chunk of salad which includes raw vegetables.

A very light breakfast, or omitting it altogether is not a good practice. A fairly complete breakfast—not heavy—is necessary. It keeps blood sugar high and one is not tempted to eat in between. It keeps the work output and mental alertness intact, which is not the case if one skips it.

Let it be noted that it takes about two weeks before reduction in weight is noticeable after the start of diet control. After this period, reduction in weight is steady.

Weight-reducing Tablets: These include thyroid tablets and those of amphetamine. Thyroid tablets have the initial effect of increasing appetite so that even though the rate of body function and consequent consumption of calories is increased, the increased intake of food neutralises this effect. Taken over a long period, they cause palpitation of the heart, restlessness, irritability and tenseness. Amphetamine and other similar drugs reduce appetite and in theory are well-suited to reducing weight. But they also cause palpitation of the heart and, if taken towards the evening, they cause insomnia.

117

Taken over long periods, the effect of reduction in appetite does not last. So both these drugs and similar ones are not of much use and should not be taken. They can prove harmful or dangerous in heart cases in particular.

Machines and Gadgets: The value of so many machines, gadgets and 'methods' of slimming used by non-medical 'experts' in the field is dubious. Weight may be lost precipitously, but it would be regained once one is off the machines.

What is necessary is to understand the mechanism of weight balance and to take measures which one can continue cheerfully as a routine.

A reduction in weight is only half the job. To maintain the reduced weight is more important and this requires a new regimen of eating habits and firm resolution.

Reduce Mental Tension

Our heart feels the effect of our emotional states and is affected by them. When someone says: "My heart felt heavy", or "My heart felt light" or "I missed a beat of my heart", it is not merely verbal expression; modern medical science is discovering that it actually can be so. A person's attitude towards life and his emotions are linked with the state of health of his heart. It has been reported in one of the studies abroad that emotional strain preceded 91 per cent of heart attacks in people between the age of 25 and 40.

Those who are given to anxieties and are ambitious and competitive and who push forward in spite of odds and obstructions, are more liable to have coronary heart disease and heart attacks. Hurrying through work constantly, is detrimental to the health of the heart. Sometime back, a comparative study was conducted on 575 male twins born in Ireland who lived for up to 20 years there and later on one of the twins shifted to Boston, U.S.A., and lived there for at least 10 years. It was found that the twin brother who shifted to the U.S.A., suffered more from coronary heart disease and heart attacks than his brother in Dublin, Ireland. This was in spite of the fact that the Dublin brother ate more fat, put on more number of hours of work in a day and had lower level of cholesterol in the blood. The important difference noted was that whereas the twin in Boston was always in a hurry in anything he did, his brother in Dublin did more physical work yet was never in too great a hurry. It seems that emotional tension increases the incidence of coronary heart disease through fat metabolism and consequent rise in the serum cholesterol levels.

Some clinical and laboratory data are available to explain the higher incidence of coronary artery disease among those who undergo greater emotional tension. According to Dr. Friedman and his colleagues (1958), a rise in serum cholesterol level was observed in accountants during the seasons of their peak activity and in medical students during the stress of examination period and during stressful interviews, in all of which the possible role of diet and exercise was excluded. These reports imply that recurrent emotional stress with consequent rise in serum cholesterol favour coronary atherosclerosis and eventual clinical coronary heart disease.

Since emotional stress is commonly associated with increased secretion of norepinephrine and epinephrine, the latter agents have been studied with regard to their effect on fat metabolism. Experimental studies in dogs indicate that epinephrine mobilises fat from its depots and causes an early rise in fatty acids and a delayed rise in cholesterol. This response is prevented by the removal of adrenal glands (adrenalectomy) but is restored when cortisone is administered before epinephrine in adrenalectomised animals. These observations indicate that both adrenal hormones and epinephrine are concerned in fat mobilisation and suggest a mechanism whereby emotional stress may raise blood fat and presumably contribute to coronary atherosclerosis.

While coronary heart disease has a multi-factorial etiology, one of the important factors that contribute to it is emotional tension. One can lessen one's chances of getting a heart attack by lessening emotional tension.

Slow down: The first essential is to slow down deliberately. One can choose between working at a lower gear without trouble and for long, or at a higher gear with trouble and with constant danger of a breakdown. "Slow and steady wins the race", is not just another maxim; it is based upon the experience of many a wise man through the ages.

Working in a relaxed mood, one can put in more number of hours and even then feel neither fatigued nor exhausted. In between the busy schedule of work, one should occasionally interrupt work just to relax.

Slowing down does not mean lessening the output. In fact, it provides more time for planning our work, and cuts down on needless activity; whatever we do is qualitatively better and the results thereof are more advantageous.

Relax your Muscles: When in a state of mental tension, the best thing for you to reduce it is to purposely relax all the muscles of the body. Let them go limp—your fists, jaws and all other muscles. Relaxed muscles relax the body.

For the same purpose, yoga advises *shavasana*, the corpse pose, in which, lying over on the back, one is to relax all the muscles of the body and lie down as if one were dead. Daily practice of it morning and evening is very useful.

Accept your Limitations: Try to accept a situation which you cannot change. It does not mean that you become apathetic. It is only that you realise your limitations. Have patience. Some problems get more entangled if one cannot practice patience.

Avoid Criticism: Learn to appreciate the good points in others. Curb your habit of criticising others. While people may say that they are broadminded about criticism, in fact, hardly anyone is. Undue criticism begets it in return.

No Tranquillisers: Tranquillisers are not the answer to one's emotional tensions. At best they lessen the emotional response to stress and anxiety. And they have very many harmful effects; they are habit-forming also.

The answer to mental tension lies in changing the habits that generate mental tension. It is important to develop a philosophy of life which generates lesser tension.

Do More of Physical Exercise

Lack of physical exercise predisposes one to getting coronary atherosclerosis. It has been found that those who do not do physical exercise possess a heart in their forties which ordinarily should belong to a person in his sixties or seventies.

Death rate from heart attacks is higher among people with sedentary occupations. Among the U.S. railroad employees, death rates were found to be 5.7 per 1,000 for clerks, 3.9 for switchmen and 2.8 for sectionmen; rates which were inversely proportionate to physical activity on the jobs. Similarly, in a study in London, it was found that there was a higher incidence of coronary heart disease in bus drivers than among other men.

Physical exercise lessens chances of a person getting heart attack; the more strenuous the exercise the lesser the heart attacks. It has lately been found that to be effective in lessening coronary atherosclerosis and heart attacks, a regular physical exercise, and once or twice a week a fairly strenuous one, is very necessary.

The Framingham data indicate that the less sedentary the occupation, the less susceptibility to sudden death. How physical activity may operate to decrease death from ischaemic heart disease or possibly atherogenesis, is not known. Beyond ameliorating hyperlipidemia by increasing caloric expenditure, no mechanism has been demonstrated. The meaning of physical activity induced increase in HDL, the anti-risk factor for ischaemic heart disease, remains mysterious.

Brisk Walks: Dr. Paul Dudley White, an eminent heart specialist, advised long walks as one of the best forms of physical exercise for the heart. To be effective, walking must be brisk. It is very good for people in the older age-groups and for those for whom the doctor does not recommend strenuous exercise, or those who have had heart attacks before. Nowadays, walking is again coming into fashion, thanks to the scarcity of petrol.

Running is very good for the heart. It exercises all the muscles of the body including those of the abdomen. If it is not convenient to run on long straight roads, one can do on-the-spot jogging in one's lawn or even in a room before a window. Care must be taken to see that the feet are raised up at least six inches from the ground.

Swimming and cycling are the other two physical exercises enjoyed by people of all the age-groups and of both of sexes.

For those who have a garden and an aptitude, gardening is a good form of physical exercise. While it keeps the body physically fit, it relaxes the mind very much.

Yogic postures (*asanas*) are in vogue these days. Learnt under the instructions of a competent teacher, they are very good for health and heart. They are not supposed to build muscles but to keep one physically and mentally sound.

Physical exercise must be done daily and regularly. Those who have not exercised their muscles for a long time, may find them sour after exercise. This is an indication that now the muscles are coming into use. If the exercise is continued, soreness passes away gradually, and a feeling of freshness and vitality sets in.

The start should be made with lighter exercise done for a shorter period. Gradually, more strenuous exercises for a longer duration can be resorted to.

After one has been doing it for quite sometime, physical exercise makes a person do more work with less expenditure of energy. That is why athletes can run for longer distances without proportionately increasing their heart rates. On the other hand, those who have flabby muscles, get breathless and tired even after light physical exertion.

For a person whose main job during the day is mental work, physical exercise is important.

Most women do not seem to take any physical exercise. But in the process of doing their daily household chores, they exert all their muscles. May be this is one of the factors that they have a low incidence of heart attacks.

However, those women who get their routine household work done by their servants and go to fashionable slimming centres may well be advised to get rid of their servants and do the work themselves; they would doubly save money, and in the process save their husbands from getting heart attacks because in the process of earning money, they have to undergo a lot of mental tension and trouble.

Physical exercise has been said to be the closest to an 'anti-ageing' pill.

Stop Smoking

Smoking increases the chances of getting a heart attack and at a younger age.

In an insurance study in the U.S.A., among policy-holders who were followed steadily and in whom smoking habits and information as to death were available, the death rate from coronary heart disease was 63 per cent higher for cigarette smokers than for non-smokers.

According to Dr. Warkerlin from the U.S.A., each year about 60,000 deaths from heart attacks in American men between 40 and 69 years of age represent deaths in excess of those to be anticipated among non-smokers.

In patients who die of other causes than coronary heart disease, advanced coronary atherosclerosis is more frequent in smokers than non-smokers. In a study involving 4,120 men, heavy cigarette smoking was associated with a three-fold increase in the incidence of severe coronary heart disease and with an increased mortality.

The immediate effect of smoking includes acceleration of heart rate, a rise in blood pressure and an increase in the amount of blood being pushed out with each beat and also increase in the work of the heart.

These effects are attributed commonly to the release of norepinephrine and epinephrine. Norepinephrine and epinephrine mobilise fatty acids from fatty tissues and raise their level in the blood. Patients who had a heart attack, experience an elevation in blood of fatty acid levels more than twice that of normal subjects. Continued smoking raises blood cholesterol as well as fatty acids, and the rise in cholesterol predisposes to coronary atherosclerosis and its complications.

An important point to note is that discontinuance of smoking lessens this risk, so much so that those who smoked previously but stopped later on, ten years after, their chances of getting a heart attack had come down to the same level as those in non-smokers.

Withdrawal Symptoms: The intensity of the initial distress produced as a result of stopping to smoke is directly proportionate to the will to stop smoking. A person who on his own accord and after fullest judgement comes to this decision, would have minimum symptoms for a few days, such as, what to do with the hands and the mouth, a certain amount of lack of concentration in work, a feeling of irritability, dry mouth, etc.

Those who are not strongly motivated, as for example, a heavy smoker who is being coaxed by his wife to stop smoking but who himself does not want to, will experience a lot of adverse symptoms. Apart from intense craving, there may be mental depression, irritability, restlessness, palpitation, sleep disturbance, difficulty in concentration, constipation, bloating in abdomen, weakness and inability to do any serious work and a host of other symptoms. The longer a person has smoked, the more his body cries out for its supply of nicotine and tobacco smoke. And when this supply is cut off, the body is bound to react.

With the first day and night safely over, a battle is won. But in many cases, the war continues. In some, a sudden craving is felt three to four days later and it increases till three to four weeks are past when it gradually abates or lessens.

How to Stop Smoking: A firm decision and the will to really stop smoking is fundamental to quitting it once and for all. If this is not there, no programme of action is going to help. Then it will be like the case of Mark Twain, who said: "It isn't difficult to quit smoking. I have done it hundreds of times."

The best method to stop smoking is to do it suddenly and completely. 'Suddenly' here does not mean on the spur of the moment. It means that you have already given a thought to the whole situation, taken some time to make the decision, and then in your mind you have fixed the best date and time for completely stopping to smoke from that time onwards.

Holidays and change of environments are the best for carrying out the resolve to give up smoking. In such a situation, one is not constantly and painfully reminded of the loss.

Another method that has been suggested for chronic smokers is to do so in planned phases. It means that the smoker resolves firmly that he is going to leave smoking. But initially he does so for a period of three weeks. He stops smoking completely and at once from a particular date and time knowing full well that he will smoke again for one or two days only after the expiry of the three week period. In such an approach, the advantage is that the smoker knows that it is a temporary loss. But, in the meanwhile, the hold of nicotine on the smoker, gradually lessens when he abstains.

Once you have stopped smoking, many temptations may come in your way to re-start it. In order to keep up your resolve, tell your friends and acquaintances about your having stopped smoking. This way, you would be binding yourself in keeping the resolve and, secondly, your friends will be cooperative with you and help you to tide over the initial period of abstinence.

As smoking depends upon the social environments, and is a highly 'contagious disease', I would advise the recent abstainers to avoid the company of smoker friends and also the situations where smoking is very frequent.

When to Resume Work after Heart Attack

That depends on many circumstances, of which your doctor, after knowing the full facts of your life, is the best judge.

1. The severity of the heart attack and how much heart muscle is damaged.

2. The speed of recovery and the absence or presence of any complications.

3. The state of the risk factor before, during and after the heart attack.

4. The kind of job you hold—sedentary work or the hard physical work.

Some types of jobs permit employees to go back part-time.

The best attitude to take in your recovery is:

1. acceptance
2. a positive outlook

When to Drive the Car

This is a tricky question.

Certainly it depends upon how severe the heart attack has been and how damaging.

Nevertheless, the attending physician decides this question. If the driving is non-taxing, perhaps, it could be resumed after six weeks. However, in heavy traffic, it may be taxing for the heart, and as such a little more delay in resuming driving, in consultation with the doctor, is advisable.

Calorie Content of Foods

Food	Quantity	Calories
Carbonated soft drinks	200 ml (1 bottle)	70
Tea, or coffee (1 teaspoon each milk & sugar)	1 cup	40 – 45
Milk: full-cream	250 gms.	160
skimmed	250 gms.	85
Beer	250 gms.	120
Brandy	30 gms.	75
Rum	50 gms.	145
Whiskey	50 gms.	135
Bread	2 Slices	100
Bread and butter	1 Slice	78
Wheat chapatties	50 gms.	100 – 125
Rice, boiled	100 gms. (boiled wt.)	70
Honey	1 tablespoon	65
Jams	1 tablespoon	55
Cream	1 tablespoon	30 – 40
Ice-cream	120 gms.	150
Butter	1 tablespoon	100
Peanut butter	1 tablespoon	85
Mayonnaise	1 tablespoon	100
Egg-whole	1 medium	75
Egg-fried	1 medium	110
Egg white, raw	1 medium	15
Egg yolk, raw	1 medium	60
Apple	1 medium	60 – 80
Apple juice, fresh	250 gms.	125
Banana	1 medium	90
Fruit cocktail canned	100 gms.	75
Grapes, fresh	100 gms.	65
Grape juice	100 gms.	70
Lemon	1 fresh	25

Food	Quantity	Calories
Orange	1 medium	60 – 70
Orange Juice, fresh	100 gms.	55
Pineapple, canned sweetened	100 gms.	90
Pineapple juice, canned	100 gms.	55
Almonds	10 nuts	75
Cashew-nuts	10 nuts	150
Vegetable soup	200 gms.	80
Vegetables (boiled)	100 gms.	35
Beans	100 gms.	80
Vegetable salad	100 gms.	85
Carrot, fresh	1 carrot, 6"	20
Cucumber	100 gms.	15
Peas, green, fresh	100 gms.	50
Tomato	1 medium	35
Tomato Juice, canned	200 gms.	35
Chicken: fried	100 gms.	250
boiled	100 gms.	200
Mutton: cooked	100 gms.	250

Calorie Allowance for Adults

Desirable wt. in Kg.	25 yrs.	45 yrs.	65 yrs.
Men			
50	2300	2050	1750
54	2400	2200	1850
59	2550	2300	1950
63	2700	2450	2050
68	2850	2550	2150
72	3000	2700	2250
77	3100	2800	2350
Women			
41	1600	1500	1250
45	1750	1600	1350
50	1900	1700	1450
54	2000	1800	1500
59	2100	1900	1600
63	2250	2050	1700
68	2350	2150	1800
72	2500	2250	1900

Calories Spent in Various Physical Activities[1]

Activity	Cal/min*	Activity	Cal/min
Standing	2.6	Badminton:	
		Recreational	5.2
Driving a car, leisurely	2.8	Competitive	10.0
Walking indoors	3.1	Basketball	6.0 – 9.0
Taking shower (with			
water at room temp.)	3.4	Tennis: Recreational	7.0
Dressing	3.4	Competitive	11.0
Cleaning windows	3.7	Soccer	9.0
Sweeping floors	3.9	Mountain climbing	10.0
Ironing clothes	4.2	Judo and karate	13.0
Gardening	4.7	Wrestling	14.0
Pick-and-shovel work	6.7		
		Swimming: Recreational	6.0
		competitive	10.0 – 12.0
Chopping wood	7.5	Dancing: Moderate	5.0
Digging earth	8.6	Walking (3.5 mph)	5.6 – 7.0
Walking up-stairs	8 – 15	up-hill (3.5 mph)	15.0
		Running	
Playing volleyball:		12 min. mile	10.0
Recreational	3.5	8 min. mile	15.0
Competitive	8.0	6 min. mile	20.0
		5 min. mile	25.0
Golf: Foursome-			
Twosome	3.7 – 5.0		
Table tennis	4.9 – 7.0		
Rowing: Recreational	5.0		
Competitive	15.0		
Cycling: 5 to 15			
miles/hr	5 – 12		
Skating: Recreation	5.0		
Vigorous	15.0		

[1]Sharkey B.J., *Physiological fitness and weight control*, Mountain Press Publishing Co., Missoula, Mont., 1974.

*Calories used per minute.

Ideal Weight for Men over 25 years

Height			Weight	
Feet	Inches	Cm.	Lbs	Kg.
5	2	157.5	118 — 129	53.5 — 58.5
5	3	160.0	121 — 133	54.9 — 60.3
5	4	162.6	124 — 136	56.2 — 61.7
5	5	165.1	127 — 139	57.6 — 63.0
5	6	167.6	130 — 143	59.0 — 64.9
5	7	170.2	134 — 147	60.8 — 66.7
5	8	172.7	138 — 152	62.6 — 68.9
5	9	175.3	142 — 156	64.4 — 70.8
5	10	177.8	146 — 160	66.2 — 72.6
5	11	180.3	150 — 165	68.0 — 74.8
6	0	182.9	154 — 170	69.9 — 77.1
6	1	185.4	158 — 175	71.7 — 79.4
6	2	188.0	162 — 180	73.5 — 81.6

Ideal Weight for Women over 25 years

Height			Weight	
Feet	Inches	Cm.	Lbs	Kg.
4	10	147.3	96 — 107	43.5 — 48.5
4	11	149.9	98 — 110	44.5 — 49.9
5	0	152.4	101 — 113	45.8 — 51.3
5	1	154.9	104 — 116	47.2 — 52.6
5	2	157.5	107 — 119	48.5 — 54.0
5	3	160.0	110 — 122	49.9 — 55.3
5	4	162.6	113 — 126	51.3 — 57.2
5	5	165.1	116 — 130	52.6 — 59.0
5	6	167.6	120 — 135	54.4 — 61.2
5	7	170.2	124 — 139	56.2 — 63.0
5	8	172.7	128 — 143	58.1 — 64.9
5	9	175.3	132 — 147	59.9 — 66.7
5	10	177.8	136 — 151	61.7 — 68.5
5	11	180.3	140 — 155	63.5 — 70.3
6	0	182.9	144 — 159	65.3 — 72.0

10

Unstable Angina

T he manifestations of ischaemic heart disease may be thought of as representing a spectrum ranging from angina pectoris at one end to acute myocardial infarction at the other. According to Braunwald and Alpert (1983), in angina pectoris, the myocardial blood supply is temporarily inadequate but there is no death of tissue, whereas myocardial infarction is, by definition, characterized by death of myocardial tissue. Some patients develop manifestations which logically place them at an intermediate, position between these two extremes, hence, the term *Intermediate Syndrome.* Included under this heading are syndromes known as acute coronary insufficiency, unstable angina, and preinfarctional angina. Unstable angina may be superimposed upon a back ground of stable exertional angina pectoris, or it may represent the first manifestation of symptomatic ischaemic heart disease.

Unstable angina pectoris may be characterized by discrete episodes of severe ischaemic chest discomfort which may come on at rest. On occasion, the discomfort begins during exertion and does not disappear with rest. The pain lasts 30 minutes or more and is of such severity that the diagnosis of myocardial infarction is considered. Although there may be in the E.C.G., ST, segment and T wave changes, myocardial infarction is ruled out by absence of both evolutionary QRS changes in the E.C.G. and diagnostic elevation of serum enzyme concentrations. Unstable angina may be superimposed upon chronic stable angina pectoris. The patient notes that his pain is precipitated by less severe exertion, comes more frequently, lasts longer, or has changed in pattern.

The specific implications of propensity to develop acute myocardial infarction, are presently debatable and the role of coronary artery bypass graft surgery in the treatment of these syndromes is thus particularly controversial. It appears that coronary bypass results, in immediate relief of unstable angina pectoris in most patients, but long-term morbidity and mortality are similar to that seen in patients treated with aggressive medical regimens. Coronary arteriography in patients with unstable angina has revealed a spectrum of morphological abnormalities ranging from severe three vessel involvement to normal coronary anatomy, indicating that the term unstable angina does not define a specific clinical entity but rather yet another pattern of presentation in the spectrum of coronary disease. Generalized statements as to either the prognosis of patients with unstable angina or the role of surgical therapy are thus not possible.

Most patients with unstable angina will stabilize with intensive medical therapy, i.e. hospitalization, bed rest, oxygen, sedation, and drug therapy with nitrates and beta-blocking agents. The adequate dose of beta-blocking agent varies from patient to patient, and increasing amounts of drug should be administered until the resting pulse rate is below 60 beats per minute. Patients with unstable angina pectoris should receive continuous E.C.G. monitoring. Given the high success rate with medical therapy (over 75 per cent) and the slightly increased risk of coronary arteriography and coronary bypass surgery in patients with unstable angina, intensive medical therapy should be the initial approach in these patients. Should such therapy be successful, as defined by the disappearance of rest pain and/or the resumption of previous activity levels, the need for early coronary arteriography with a view toward emergency surgery is obviated. The question of coronary arteriography and coronary bypass graft surgery may then be considered on an elective basis as it would be in any patient with chronic stable coronary artery disease.

On the other hand, if unstable angina persists despite intensive, medical therapy, an advisable course is to carry out coronary arteriography and, if the anatomy is suitable, revascularization surgery.

The exercise test is probably unusually hazardous and hence contraindicated in patients with unstable angina pectoris and patients who have suffered acute myocardial infarction during the preceding few weeks.

11

Angina Pectoris

A ngina pectoris is a condition wherein a patient gets recurrent attacks of pain or oppression behind the sternum (chest bone), radiating to the region of the heart and to the left arm, precipitated usually by physical exertion and relieved on resting. Angina means strangulation; pectoris means 'of the chest'. This is a manifestation of atherosclerosis of the coronary arteries.

Approximately four-fifths of all patients with angina pectoris are men. The typical patient is in his fifties or early sixties.

Characteristics of Anginal Pain

This pain is usually dull and diffuse, yet it has a special characteristic: it gives a feeling of strangling, constricting, pressing, like a vise or tight band around the chest, with occasionally a feeling as if the person is going to pass away. It compels the patient to remain as quiet as possible.

When the pain radiates to the left arm, it does not necessarily move in a continuous line from the chest to the arm; often there is no geographic contiguity between the pain in the arm and the pain in the chest; they merely occur together. Sometimes, the pain is localised to the sternal region and affects the arm or other parts only when it is severe or protracted. The pain may reach the shoulder and upper arm and then skip to the wrist, or it may radiate to the wrist and fingers alone without involving any other portion of the left arm. It usually occurs along the inner side of the arm, the hand and the little finger.

When severe, the pain may spread to both shoulders or even to both upper arms. The pain may extend to the collar bone, the clavicle, lower neck or throat, jaw and teeth, especially on the left side. Frequently, the sensation in the arms, wrist or hands is described as a numbness or weakness, less commonly as tingling.

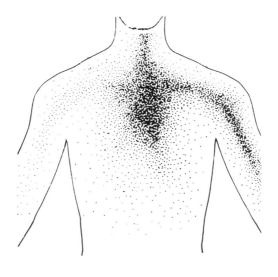

Fig. 15   Radiation of Pain

This pain usually lasts only a few minutes, but the patient overestimates the duration. Such attacks generally subside after a minute or two if the patient rests immediately when the pain begins.

These attacks of pain vary greatly in frequency. Many patients, having learned the maximal activity in which they can indulge without pain, avoid pain completely for long periods by restricting physical exertion below the critical point. Some patients suffer a single paroxysm of pain early in the day, usually on walking, after which they are able to carry on normal activity or even relatively strenuous work without symptoms. Others have only occasional seizures at intervals of days, weeks, or months—the intervals depending, to some extent, on avoidance of the factors which excite their attacks. Still other patients experience numerous seizures each day, often without cause, or after some slight activity or emotional experience, even after simple daily chores.

Besides pain, the patient may complain of "inability to breathe" though it is not breathlessness. Belching is common and passage of flatus or desire to pass urine, occurs occasionally at the end of the attack.

Relation to Physical Exertion

Physical exertion is by far the most frequent and most significant precipitating cause of anginal pain. Often a patient gets it for the first time while running for a bus on his way to work or while walking up a slight incline. From then on, the pain recurs whenever he runs or walks uphill or even on a level beyond a limited distance.

Walking outdoors is the commonest form of bodily exertion, producing the pain. Cold and wind, a preceding meal and a sense of hurry increases its probability. Some patients have to stop in between while walking.

The pain or discomfort comes on during physical or emotional stress, anger, fright, hurrying or sexual activity. Manual chores which have been performed for many years may be well tolerated, whereas unfamiliar tasks requiring comparable effort may cause angina.

Cause of Pain

The underlying cause of angina pectoris is the narrowing of the coronary arteries due to atherosclerosis. Lesser blood flows through them and hence less oxygen is supplied to the heart muscle. The sensation of pain is caused by the production and collection of unoxidised metabolic products in the heart muscle which in turn stimulate the numerous sensory nerves surrounding the coronary arteries. From there it is conducted via nervous pathways to the area where it is felt.

Pain in the chest following bodily exertion is due to the increased work of the heart which requires more oxygen, but this cannot be supplied through the narrowed arteries. After taking a heavy meal, digestion, like exercise, increases the work of the heart. Exposure to cold also increases workload of the heart. So is the case with emotional tension.

The pain is transitory in nature, lasting as long as the extra demands of the heart persist; once the patient rests, and there is no need of extra blood to the heart muscle, the symptoms disappear.

Diagnosis

The essential features of angina pectoris are:
1. the paroxysmal occurrence of the pain;
2. its brief duration;
3. its characteristic location, radiation and quality;
4. its precipitation by effort and relief by rest.

The occurrence of chest pain during strong emotional experiences, with relief when the emotional reaction subsides, is likewise characteristic of angina pectoris.

Radiation to the left shoulder, arm and wrist or both arms is usually confirmatory of angina pectoris, but not essential for the diagnosis. The strangling, constricting or compressing quality of the pain and the occasional association of the feeling of passing away are valuable diagnostic features.

Because of the wide distribution of anginal pain, it may be mistaken for pain due to diseases of other structures, such as the gall-bladder, pancreas, stomach, intestines, muscles and bones about the chest and left shoulder and even teeth. Yet proper physical examination and laboratory tests provide the necessary clues.

When the essential symptomatic criteria are satisfied, the diagnosis of angina pectoris may be made with certainty even in the absence of objective findings. A suspected diagnosis of angina pectoris may be supported by finding hypertension, significant heart enlargement, or E.C.G. abronmalitics during an attack.

Stress Test

If absent before, the E.C.G. changes can be brought about in a patient of angina pectoris by making him take physical exercise. This measures the capacbility of the coronary circulation to augment coronary blood flow in response to increased myocardial oxygen demands.

The most widely used test in the diagnosis of ischaemic heart disease involves recording the 12-lead E.C.G. before, during and after exercise on a treadmill or using a bicycle ergometer. The patient undergoes a standardized incremental increase in extenal workload while the E.C.G., symptoms, and arm blood pressure are continuously monitored. The test is usually symptom-limited, and is discontinued with the onset of chest discomfort, severe shortness of breath, dizziness, fatique, ST-segment depression of greater than 2 mm, a fall in systolic blood pressure exceeding 15 mm Hg, or the development of ventricular tachycardia or arrhythmia.

This test seeks to establish the relationship between chest discomfort and the typical electrocardiographic signs of myocardial ischaemia. The rate of false-positive diagnosis is approximately 15 per cent and an approximately equal percentage of patients with severe, multi-vessel coronary artery block will not have a positive test (false negative).

Negative exercise tests in which the target heart rate (85 per cent of maximal heart rate for age and sex) is not achieved, are considered to be non-diagnostic.

A positive exercise result indicates the likelihood of coronary artery disease in 98 per cent in patients with typical angina pectoris, 88 per cent in those with atypical chest pain, 44 per cent in those patients with non-anginal chest pain and 33 per cent in asymptomatic persons.

The physician should be present throughout the exercise test and it is important to measure total duration of exercise, the external work performed, and the internal cardiac work performed, as represented by the heart rate—blood pressure product with the time to the onset of ischaemic ST-segment change and chest discomfort. It is also important to note the depth of the ST-segment depression and the time for recovery of these electrocardiographic changes.

Because the risks of exercise testing are small but real, equipment for resuscitation should be available. The risks are estimated at one fatality and two non-fatal complication per 10,000 tests.

Prognosis

Atherosclerosis of the coronary arteries is a gradually progressive process, so that with the passage of time, more and more narrowing occurs.

A patient who gets attacks of angina pectoris is more liable to get heart attack. He is also liable to get minor or major brain strokes because atherosclerosis involves arteries of the brain also.

There may not be, however, any immediate danger. Most patients live at least 5 to 10 years after the onset of this disease; some patients have survived up to 20 years.

A history of angina pectoris and heart attack in many members of the family, especially in the parents, with death at an early age, bespeaks an unfavourable course. As a general rule, the earlier the onset of angina, the lower the age at death. Marked hypertension or heart enlargement, previous heart attacks and heart failure or diabetes are among the associated findings which worsen the prognosis.

Angina pectoris may disappear for long periods of time or permanently, even after it has been present for months or years. This may be due to the development of the increased collateral circulation.

Angina Decubitus

The term angina decubitus has been applied to the variant of angina pectoris which develops while the patient is in the recumbent position. The patient may report that he is awakened at night by a sensation which is similar to his exertional pain. The syndrome of angina decubitus is similar to that of paroxysmal nocturnal dyspnoea, and dyspnoea actually often accompanies the chest discomfort. It is postulated, but not proved that the pathophysiolgy is also similar and that angina decubitus is a form of left ventricular failure precipitated by the expansion of the intrathoracic blood volume which occurs with recumbency and which may increase myocardial oxygen requirements. Elevation of systemic arterial blood pressure has been demonstrated to precede attacks of pain in some instances and may be another precipitating factor. Dreaming has also been implicated in the pathogenesis of this relatively unusual variant of angina.

Variant Angina or Prinzmetal's Angina

More recently, a distinctive subset of this condition has been recognized, known as variant angina or Prinzmetal's angina. This form is characterized by the development of the pain at rest, and sometimes is associated with ventricular arrhythmias. In contrast to effort angina with its typical depression of the ST segment in the E.C.G., Prinzmetals' angina typically exhibits ST segment elevations.

The pain is thought to arise from some sudden and transient imbalance between myocardial needs and coronary flow. Almost invariably, atherosclerosis of the coronary arteries, usually moderately severe, underlies such attacks.

Variant angina represents transmural ischaemia often due to spasm of one of the major coronary arteries.

Treatment of Angina

General Measures : The term management is more appropriate than treatment with reference to angina pectoris, because far more is required than the prescription of a drug or the recommendation of operation. The patient must be evaluated with particular reference to the interaction between his disease and life pattern. The physical and emotional stresses which precipitate pain and the pleasurable activities prohibited by angina must be identified.

The patient must be made to realize that long useful lie is possible even though he has angina pectoris.

Patients of angina pectoris soon themselves come to learn that reducing the speed of walking and the speed of doing other routine chores lessens the frequency of attacks. Running for buses is strictly forbidden for them. Walking immediately after meals is prohibited as it is liable to bring on an attack. Sudden and unusual forms of physical exertion should be avoided. Heavy meals, emotional outbursts, prolonged conversation on controversial subjects either face to face or even on telephone, straining at stools, must be avoided. Participating in or watching games which excite temper should be avoided.

Immediately after the first attack of angina pectoris, rest in bed or great limitation of movement for two weeks is advisable. This is to avoid any risk of heart attack. If the attacks recur, they do not require the patient to rest in bed, but if the attacks occur frequently, and even with slight bodily exertion, they may compel the patient to take rest. The patient is well advised to call his physician in case the pain of an attack persists for more than 15 minutes or if it is more intense and different from the pain of previous attacks.

A patient of angina pectoris needs to re-orient his life and leisure. Long hours of work causing fatigue have to be avoided. Afternoon rest is must. If he is in a job requiring moderately severe physical exertion or requiring precision work before a machine, he should change to a lighter duty which avoids endangering his own or other persons' lives.

His holiday or vacation programme should be such as gives physical and mental rest. Going to mountains in summer needs care and consideration; theoretically, it is not advisable as the air on the high mountains has less oxygen to breathe in and it makes the heart work harder; moreover, ups and downs in the mountains are physically more tiring. But, if things can be arranged so that the patient lives on the hills for some weeks in the summer, without doing any extra physical exertion and is certain to get mental rest away from the tiring routine, he may be advised by his family doctor to go to the hills.

The diet should aim at two things:
1. Trying to check the progress of atherosclerosis, and
2. Not to put extra burden on the heart to digest it.

If the patient is overweight, his diet has to be such as reduces the weight. Usually, a low calorie diet should be taken, dividing the total amount eaten into more number of times and eating less quantity at a time. Large meals should be strictly avoided.

Smoking should be stopped completely, and moderation used in taking tea and coffee. An occasional peg of whiskey causes no, harm—if one is fond of drinks.

If diabetes is present which needs the use of drugs or injections to lower blood sugar, care should be taken to avoid too much lowering of blood sugar as it leads to the onset of anginal pain.

Relief of Pain : If hypertension is present, drug therapy should be instituted so as to bring it under control.

For immediate relief of pain and to avoid having pain in a situation where a little over-exertion cannot be avoided, different types of nitrites are used whose action is supposed to last for a shorter or longer duration. However, under no circumstances should nitrites be taken to perform some unusual strenuous activity which is likely to cause harm. They are, of course, unnecessary when the pain is very mild and of brief duration.

Nitrites are said to dilate the coronary arteries and to increase coronary blood flow supplying more oxygen to the heart muscle.

Nitroglycerin is the drug of choice. It is cheap and convenient to take and it acts rapidly. It comes in tablets which the patient puts under his tongue to dissolve. If the tablets are not readily soluble they may be inert or their action delayed. Usually they do not lose their effectiveness if kept for long. These tablets come in 1/100th, 1/200th and 1/400th of a gram; 1/100th gram tablet is usually sufficient. However, to begin with, the patient should take 1/200th gram tablet which often suffices and is less likely to induce uncomfortable side actions. Its action is noticeable in 1 to 2 minutes and continues for 15 minutes to an hour. In most cases, the relief is striking as well as prompt. Often, however, it may be accompanied by mild fulness, warmth or throbbing in the head. For such patients, 1/400th gram tablets may be effective and more tolerable. With continued use of the drug, the side-effects usually diminish in severity or disappear. Immediately after taking the tablet, the patient should sit down or find some support. Nitroglycerin should not be taken for those attacks which are known to subside promptly with a brief period of rest. Since the pain disappears rapidly and spontaneously, there is no need for the patient to suffer any unpleasant side actions of the drug.

Patients with angina should be instructed to take the medication to relieve an attack and also in anticipation of stress which is likely to induce angina. A flight of stairs, a walk up a hill or sexual intercourse may produce pain consistently, but often the pain can be prevented by the anticipatory use of nitroglycerin. The value of this prophylactic use of drug cannot be over-emphasized.

If nitroglycerin produces neither relief of pain nor a headache, nor a slight sensation of burning at the sublingual site of absorption, the preparation may be inactive, and a fresh supply should be obtained.

If the patient does not experience relief after the first dose of nitroglycerin, he may take a second, or even a third, but should be instructed not to continue to take the medication if the first few doses prove unsuccessful. If pain continues despite nitroglycerin, the patient should consult his physician, or report promptly to a hospital emergency room for evaluation for the possibility of an acute myocardial infarction.

Amylnitrite acts even more rapidly in 10 to 15 seconds but its action lasts only for several minutes. It is administered in small glass pearls or ampoules which must be crushed in a handkerchief and inhaled. Its disadvantages are its expense, inconvenience in carrying and administration, and the distinctive odour which calls undesirable attention to the patient when it is taken in the presence of others. Its unpleasant side actions are similar to those of nitroglycerin.

Longer-acting nitrites are designed to provide the same effect as nitroglycerin or amylnitrite but for a prolonged and sustained duration. With them it is hoped that anginal attacks can be prevented, or at least reduced in number and severity. The action of these nitrites is dependent on the continued release of nitrites.

Unfortunately, none of the long-acting nitrites is as effective as nitroglycerin in the relief of angina pectoris. However, several of these preparations are useful in prolongging the time interval between attacks, and, hence, in reducing the amount of nitroglycerin which has to be taken as therapy for acute attacks.

Preparations which are chewed or taken sublingually and therefore depend upon absorption through the mucous membranes are more effective than those that are simply swallowed. If one preparation is ineffective, another should be tried, as many patients find one preparation more effective than others. There is marked variation among patients in the dose required to produce a result, especially in the preparations to be swallowed, just as there is variation in the dose of nitrolycerin required for relief of an acute attack. The dosage of the long-acting agent should be increased gradually until either a therapeutic or toxic effect is encountered. It may be taken on a regular basis every few hours by patients with frequent anginal attacks, in addition to being taken in anticipation of events known to provoke angina.

Nitroglycerin ointment applied to the chest can be utilized as a slow-release preparation which is especially useful in the treatment of angina decubitus. An application of ointment at bedtime may give the patient a night's sleep which had not been possible before.

Sedatives and tranquilisers are among the most widely prescribed drugs. They include phenobarbitone, bromides, chloral hydrate and a host of others available in the market. Their benefit in angina pectoris applies only indirectly, in so far as they serve to reduce emotional tension.

Patient of angina pectoris should avoid taking injections of adrenaline, and even tablets which contain ephedrine or other similar drugs or which increase heart rate and blood pressure.

Newer Drugs : The beta-adrenergic blocking agents, such as propranolol, represent a useful addition to the pharmacological treatment of angina pectoris. The effects of these drugs are most apparent during exercise when they decrease cardiac output and heart rate and thus work load on the heart. Propranolol is usually given in an initial dose of 40 mg a day and increased if necessary. A pulse rate of 45 per minute or less and clinical evidence of impairment of left ventricular function or heart failure are contraindications to giving beta blocking drugs.

Another new group of drugs to treat angina is the calcium channel blockers (nifedipine, verapamil, diltiazem). Widely used in Europe for several years, these have recently been used in India. Because of their patent coronary vasodilatory properties, they have proved to be extremely useful in the treatment of Prinzmetals' angina and other forms of angina in which coronary spasm plays a role. In addition, calcium channel blockers reduce myocardial oxygen demands by reducing arterial pressure and myocardial contractibility and are useful in the treatment of chronic stable angina. They can be used together with beta-blockers and nitrites and produce an additive effect. However, when such combination treatment is employed, it is important to follow the patient carefully to ensure that hypertension and heart failure do not occur.

Every Chest Pain is not Heart Attack

With the increasing incidence of heart attacks, some people have become over-conscious of the condition so that to them any pain in the chest raises doubts in their minds whether it could be a heart attack.

Let us try to differentiate the pain due to an angina pectoris and heart attack from other conditions in which pain in the chest occurs as one of the symptoms.

The pain of angina pectoris, as described already, starts after physical exertion or an emotional upset in the region behind the sterum. It is a dull pain which may radiate to the left arm towards the little finger. It has a constricting quality and may be accompanied by a feeling as if one is going to pass away. It is relieved soon after taking rest or after taking a nitrite tablet. This pain is only transitory, lasting for not less than a minute and usually not more than 15 minutes.

The pain of heart attack is more prolonged. It is usually not initiated by any physical exertion. It may be accompanied by sweating and breathlessness. The patient may become unconscious and fall down. His pulse may become rapid and blood pressure low. The pain lasts several hours, and is relieved, to an extent, after injection of morphine or pethidine.

Cardiac Neurosis: A dull ache, or sharp, sticking or stabbing pain in the region of the heart or in the left breast occurs frequently in neurotic persons. In addition, there is often a complaint of excessive fatigability, palpitation, diffuse pains in different parts of the body and difficulty in taking a deep breath characterised objectively by sighing respiration. In addition to the difference in site and character of the pain, it occurs at rest as well as with angina effort.

Discomfort behind Sternum due to Fatigue: Sometimes

discomfort is felt behind the sternum or over the heart in the left chest. This comes on after prolonged work and subsequent fatigue, but is not promptly relieved by rest. Sometimes pain in the front of the chest occurs only or especially when the patient sits down and relaxes after some strenuous work or after a hard day. This has nothing to do with angina pectoris.

Abdominal Conditions: The error of diagnosing heart attack as acute indigestion is becoming less common. On the other hand, there is a growing tendency to err in the opposite direction: labelling an episode of indigestion as heart attack.

A definite diagnosis of heart attack should be made only if the clinical features, the E.C.G. changes or both are sufficiently characteristic.

On the other hand, a history of some indiscretion in diet, loose motions, vomiting, etc. are points towards abdominal upset.

The pain due to peptic ulcer, inflammation of or stones in the gall-bladder, acute inflammation of the pancreas, acute abdominal obstruction or even acute appendicitis may simulate a heart attack.

The pain due to stomach and duodenal ulcer is usually situated in the region just below the sternum. It has a burning or boring quality, is unrelated to effort and occurs usually one to four hours after meals. The pain due to an ulcer is ordinarily rapidly relieved by alkalies and milk.

Inflammation of the gall-bladder or stones in the gall-bladder occur more often in women who are in the middle-age group and are rather obese. Aggravation of symptoms after a fatty meal; physical examination and an X-ray of the abdomen confirm the diagnosis.

The pain due to acute inflammation of the pancreas radiates both towards the front as well as the back. This pain is difficult to differentiate from pain due to heart attack. Laboratory investigation of the enzymes liberated from the pancreas into the blood which subsequently are excreted in the urine, and an E.C.G. help in establishing the diagnosis.

Lung Conditions: Pulmonary embolism in which an embolus lodges in an artery of the lung, thereby blocking flow of blood in it, produces symptoms of acute pain in the chest, cough and sometimes spitting of blood in the sputum. Pulmonary embolism may look like a heart attack. E.C.G. and X-ray of the chest help in differentiating these two conditions.

Pain in the chest and fever are also the symptoms of pericarditis, i.e. inflammation of the outer covering of the heart, the pericardium. Differentiation in diagnosis depends on E.C.G. changes. Sometimes a heart attack is accompanied by pericarditis when the heart infarct touches the inner surface of the pericardium.

Rupture of the lung into the pleura called spontaneous pneumothorax is distinguished by absence of E.C.G. changes of heart attack. This condition produces distinctive physical and X-ray findings of the presence of air in the pleura.

Rupture of the lung into the aorta causing bleeding between two layers of its wall—the condition being called dissecting aneurysm of the aorta—occurs predominantly among males between the ages of 40 and 70 who have pre-existing high blood pressure—the sort of patients in whom heart attack also occurs more commonly. The diagnosis is strongly suggested by the history of thoracic or upper abdominal pain which from the onset or shortly thereafter is situated in the back, by its severity and tearing quality, by its very acute onset without any warning symptoms, by its maximal intensity at the very onset and by its frequent radiation or migration to involve the neck, shoulders, lumber or costo-vertebral regions, groins, hips or lower extremity.

The maintenance of the usually elevated blood pressure and absence of E.C.G. changes of heart attack are the important features which differentiate dissecting aneurysm from heart attack.

Rib and Joint Conditions: Pain may be associated with bones and joints of the ribs and the spine. Of particular interest is pain due to an inflammation present at the junction of a rib with its cartilage on either side near the upper part of the sternum. This condition is called Tietze's syndrome. This pain is continuous and increases in intensity on applying pressure over the inflammed area. There may be a swelling over the inflammed region.

An often unrecognised cause of pain, referred to the region of the heart and left arm is due to sprain or strain in the muscle and ligaments about the lower neck and upper thoracic spine. Stiff neck may have been the first symptom. Local examination of the part, helps in establishing diagnosis.

Sometimes osteoarthritis of the upper throacic spine or lesions of the spinal cord or nerve roots produce shooting pain over the region of the heart. This pain occurs in bandlike zones involving the front and back of the chest corresponding to the involved nerve segments. This pain is not related to general body effort but is induced by motions of the spinal column or by factors increasing intraspinal pressure such as coughing and sneezing.

Occasionally, pain in the left upper arm and over the region of the heart is due to compression of the nerves by a cervical rib. This pain is sharp or aching and often radiates to the fourth and fifth fingers. It may be associated with numbness and tingling. X-ray of the chest bones and a complete neurological examination helps in establishing diagnosis.

Thus we see that pain in the chest occurs in diverse conditions. It is not very difficult to establish its true identity. A doctor with his clinical experience and with the help of X-ray, E.C.G. and other relevant laboratory tests can establish the true nature of the disease.

Brain Strokes

People who are liable to get heart attack or angina, are also liable to get brain stroke. Diabetics, and in particular, women diabetics, are especially susceptible to get both the conditions.

The basic cause of these strokes is atherosclerosis of the blood vessels of the brain. Atherosclerosis not only involves the coronary arteries giving rise to heart attacks or anginal pain, but it involves arteries in other parts of the body, more significant of which are the arteries that supply oxygen to the brain. Narrowing of the arteries of brain (as in the case of the heart) occurs gradually over the years and decades. The process is accelerated in patients who are diabetic and those who have high blood pressure.

When thrombosis develops in one of the narrowed blood vessels in the brain, changes similar to those of cardiac infarction occur in the brain. There is the central area in which necrosis occurs because of the lack of blood and oxygen. Around this area of necrosis, swelling (oedema) occurs which involves a larger part of the brain.

Gradually, over the days, this swelling lessens and finer functions return which are altered not because of necrosis but due to swelling of the brain only In a matter of week or a fortnight, the patient feels that he is better. The area bereft of blood becomes narrowed down by collateral flow from surrounding regions, which speeds recovery of function.

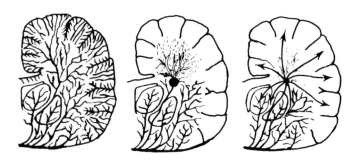

Fig. 16   Blocking of Cerebral Artery and its Effect on the Peripheral Branches

An ischaemic infarction of the brain is not demonstrable on gross examination with any certainty until after about 6 to 12 hours of survival. The earliest change is a slight discoloration and softening of the affected area, so that gray matter takes on a muddy colour and the white matter loses its normal fine grained appearance. Within 48 to 72 hours necrosis is well established and there is disintegration of the ischaemic area with swelling around it. Eventually if the lesion is of sufficient size, there is liquefaction and cyst formation, the cyst being traversed by the blood vessels.

Paralytic stroke may as well be due to a rupture in a hardened and sclerosed blood vessel. The onset of symptoms may be slow but they progress rapidly and soon the patient may be in deep coma from which he may not be brought back.

Symptoms

The symptoms depend upon the site and nature of the vascular lesion. It may cause sudden death, if the blocked artery supplied blood to an area of the brain which is vital to life. There may be paralysis on one side of the body (hemiplegia) and loss of speech or difficulty in formulating speech. The lesion in the brain is on the

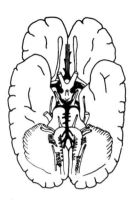

Fig. 17   Under-surface of the Brain showing Arterial system.

side opposite to that of paralysis of the limbs; this is because the brain nerve fibres cross over before they supply the limbs. Furthermore, the speech centre is located on the left side of the brain; so if there is a lesion there, there is loss of speech as well as hemiplegia of the right side.

In a patient who becomes unconscious after the stroke, it may be observed that his eyes are deviated to one side, the pupils of the eyes are unequal in size or are contracted and they do not respond to light. In proportion to the severity of disturbance, respiration tends to be hurried, noisy and stertorous. Swallowing is often impossible; there is no control over passing urine or retention may occur. Reflexes tend to be lost on the side of the paralysis.

The severity of the lesion can be judged from the depth of coma, from the degree of which the patient responds to any form of stimulation and from the signs of failure of respiration.

Hemiplegia may completely recover, but unless improvement begins early and progresses rapidly, it is not likely to be complete. The restoration of movements follow a certain order: deviation of the tongue and facial asymmetry clears up early; next the leg begins to recover, and finally and, often very incompletely, the arm. The return of movements in the limbs is selective. In both upper and

151

lower limbs, movement at the proximal joints recover first and most completely. The fine skilled movements of the hands and fingers are frequently lost for ever.

Diagnosis

It is very difficult indeed to tell at the time of the event if a stroke is the result of thrombosis or haemorrhage. Lumber puncture and examination of the cerebrospinal fluid help in diagnosis. The cerebrospinal fluid in recent thrombosis is never found to contain blood, but a little later, it is often coloured yellow or yellowish brown from escape of changed blood pigments, when the lesion has reached the surface of the convexity or the surface of the ventricle. In case of haemorrhage, it contains blood within a very short time of the onset.

Computerized tomography of the brain (CT scan) has proved a most valuable tool for the diagnosis of stroke. Although CT may be normal in the initial days after infarction, a focal area of decreased density rapidly follows, as the infarct liquefies. When the patient is seen early in the course of atherosclerotic thrombosis, it is extremely difficult to give an immediate prognosis. No rules have yet been laid down which allow one to predict its course. A mild paralysis today may become disastrous hemiplegia tomorrow, or the patient's condition may only worsen temporarily for a day or two. The course of the defect is so often progressive that a cautious attitude on the part of the physician is justified in what appears to be a mild stroke.

Treatment

Complete physical examination to assess the loss of function is the first essential. The next is to find out any other accompanying disease or a complication that has set in after the stroke, for example, retention of urine. The drugs prescribed depend upon the assessment of the individual patient. Maintenance of a steady but a little higher than normal blood pressure is essential. Proper hygienic cleaning of the patient and movement of the limbs is essential.

When hemiplegia has become established, the patient should be mobilised early, sitting in a chair as soon as possible. When his general condition permits, the affected limbs must be put through the full range of active and passive movements twice each day. When not being exercised, muscles which may contract should be stretched on a padded wire frame. Sustained improvement depends on attention to details of general management of bowel and bladder, and upon encouragement of the use of every function as it returns in the aphasic patient, speech therapy should await return of the function of speech to justify its use.

Transient Ischaemic Attacks

Sixty per cent of the cases of thrombotic strokes are preceded by transient ischaemic attack. The risk of stroke in the population of cases experiencing transient ischaemic attack is 6 to 7 per cent the first year, and the 5-year cumulative risk reaches an alarming 35 to 50 per cent.

Attention is directed to these attacks for the reason that their treatment (the administering of anticoagulant drugs or performing surgical endarterectomy at the stage of prodromal symptoms) may prevent a disastrous stroke. There would seem to be little doubt that they are due to transient focal ischaemia, and they might be referred to as temporary strokes which fortunately reverse themselves. Corresponding to the higher incidence of atherosclerosis in hypertension and in the male population, about two-thirds of all patients with trasient ischaemic attacks are hypertensive and/or men.

Clinical Picture: Thrombosis of virtually any cerbral or cerebellar artery, deep or superficial, can be associated with transient ischaemic attacks. Trasient ischaemic attacks last from a few up to 24 hours, the most common duration being a few seconds up to 5 to 10 minutes. It is uncommon for recurrent discrete attacks to last more than 30 minutes. There may be only a few attacks or several hundred. Between attacks the neurologic examination may disclose no abnormalities. A stroke may ensue after the second episode or may be postponed until hundreds of attacks have occured over a period of weeks or months. The neurologic features of the transient episode indicate the territory of the artery involved.

Generalised Atherosclerosis of the Brain Arteries

Generalised narrowing of arteries of the brain and their branches causes a more widespread damage in the brain. The accumulative effect of narrowing and blockage of the blood vessels is degeneration of the brain so that the patient's range of interest becomes reduced and intellectual activities restricted. Memory for recent events becomes faulty, while that for events long past remains unimpaired. Confusion is liable to occur and the patient becomes unable to adapt himself to new circumstances and is obstinately conservatie. Emotional control becomes impaired. Previously existing tendencies to anxiety, or depression may become exaggerated. The physical symptoms take the form of a slowly developing muscular rigidity, the face becomes set, movements become less free, and in walking the step becomes gradually shortened and it may be only a few inches.

Treatment is only symptomatic; the patient should be kept up and about as long as possible.

Coronary Bypass Surgery in India

Coronary bypass surgery (CBS) is at present performed in different centres in India. The following are the more important amongst them:

New Delhi

All India Institute of Medical Sciences

G.B. Pant Hospital

Batra Hospital (started late)

Bombay

Jaslok Hospital

Beach Candy Hospital

KEM College

Madras

Apollo Hospital

Vellore

Christian Medical College (CMC)

Paranbur

Railway Hospital

At present, the maximum number of CBS operations are being done at the Apollo Hospital—750 to 1000 a year.

Are you fit enough to benefit from Physical Exercise

Before embarking on any physical exercise programme you should check how fit you are.

A relatively simple and safe way of doing this is to measure your pulse rate. The first thing you want to know is the rate while the body is at rest, so the measurement should be taken first thing in the morning before the rate can be affected by exertion, tension, nicotine, coffee, tea or alcohol.

Normal Pulse Rate

Pulse rates vary, but 70 to 85 beats per minute is the average for men and 75 to 90 beats is the average for women.

The Danger Zone

Whatever your sex, if your resting pulse rate is in the nineties you are unfit, and if it is over 100 you have cause for concern and should seek an immediate check-up.

Once you have established that you are reasonably fit, you must check on the safe maximum pulse rates you can achieve during exercise.

Check Your Fitness Level

Even without taking your pulse, it is easy to get an idea of how fit you are by completing the checklist below. Put a tick (✓) in the box if your answer is yes.

1. You can feel your heart thumping after climbing a few flights of stairs. ☐
2. You are left gasping for breath even after running a short distance only. ☐
3. It is a great effort to bend and tie your shoelaces. ☐
4. You are tired out after carrying two bags of shopping for about a kilometre. ☐
5. You avoid physical effort, if you possibly can. ☐

If you have ticked any of the above and are aged under 50 years, you probably would benefit from more exercise.

How To Take Your Own Pulse

What you are actually feeling when you take your pulse is the waves of blood travelling from the heart along a main artery. The pulse is normally felt at the wrist, because the beat is strong and in an easily accessible place, but pulses can be felt in many other parts of the body also, such as the neck.

The 'Resting Pulse'

To take your pulse, use a watch that shows seconds.

1. Hold the wrist with your right hand (see diagram) and move the first two fingers of your right hand until you can feel the pulse just under your thumb on the left wrist.

2. Count the number of beats that occur during a sixty second interval.

Multiply the number of beats by two to get the number of beats per minute.

To get the 'resting pulse' you should do this first thing in the morning, while sitting in a relaxed position.

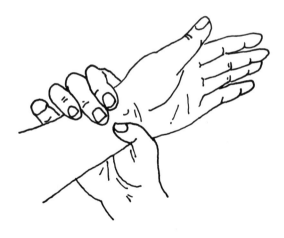

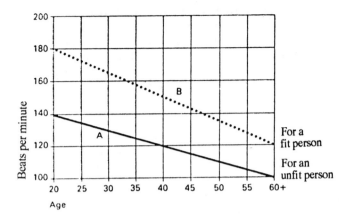

Safe Maximum Pulse Rate During Exercise

This depends on two things: your age and your current level of fitness.

For a fit person, the heart can beat at a maximum of about 200 beats per minute at age 20, but at only about 150 beats at age 70. When you are exerting yourself your pulse rate should not rise above 75% of your maximum.

A useful and a safe formula for calculating the ideal rate for you is:

200 minus your age minus another 40 if you are very unfit. Thus for an unfit 50-year-old the rate would be: 200—50—40—110 beats/minute.

The graph gives you at a glance estimate of the approximate desireable rates during exercise for different ages and levels of fitness.

Desirable Life Style Changes

1. Talk slower, interrupt less, less emphasis in talking.

2. Reflect and paraphrase more. Focus full attention on other person(s).

3. Less abrupt fidgeting and jiggling. Smile and laugh more: look for the humour in things.

4. Practise waiting with more patience (e.g., in bank, restaurant, post office, supermarket, department store, traffic jam); use waiting time to reflect.

5. Spend time physically relaxing - 20 minutes a day.

6. Reduce TV watching of violent, highly competitive or disturbing events.

7. Do not take on new or additional tasks without at least reducing current tasks (no 'add-ons').

8. Speak more often with neighbours; take time to be friendly.

9. Drive more slowly and stay in the right lane.

10. Minimize heavy or large meals with foods high in fats.

11. Eat more often during the day instead of having one meal at the end of the day.

12. Comply with prescribed medication.

Dear Reader,

Welcome to the world of **Orient Paperbacks**—India's largest selling paperbacks in English. We hope you have enjoyed reading this book and would want to know more about **Orient Paperbacks.**

There are more than 700 **Orient Paperbacks** on a variety of subjects to entertain and inform you. The list of authors published in **Orient Paperbacks** includes, amongst others, distinguished and well-known names as Dr. S. Radhakrishnan, R.K. Narayan, Raja Rao, Manohar Malgonkar, Khushwant Singh, Anita Desai, Kamala Das, Dr. O.P. Jaggi, H.K. Bakhru, Norman Vincent Peale, Robert Schuller, Windy Dryden, Paul Hauck and Sasthi Brata. **Orient Paperbacks** truly represent the best of Indian writing in English today.

We would be happy to keep you continuously informed of the new titles and programmes of **Orient Paperbacks** through our monthly newsletter, **Orient Literary Review.** Send in your name and full address to us today. We will start sending you **Orient Literary Review** completely free of cost.

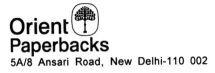